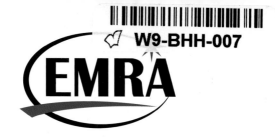

2015 EMRA / AIRWAY•CAM

Fundamentals of Airway Management

3rd Edition

Richard M. Levitan, MD, FACEP

AIRWAY•CAM Technologies, Inc.

PUBLISHER
Emergency Medicine Residents' Association
1125 Executive Circle, Irving, TX 75038-2522
972.550.0920
www.emra.org

EMRA STAFF
Cathey Wise, Executive Director
Leah Stefanini, Meetings & Advertising Manager
Linda Baker, Marketing & Operations Manager
Chalyce Bland, Project Coordinator
Valerie Hunt, Managing Editor

Disclaimer
This handbook is intended as a general guide to patient care only.
It is not intended to replace formal training. The publisher, author,
editors, and sponsoring organizations specifically disclaim any
liability for any omissions or errors found in this handbook, for
appropriate use, or treatment errors.

ISBN 978-1-929854-39-4

EMRA Board of Directors

Author

Dr. Rich Levitan was in the first class of emergency medicine residents at Bellevue Hospital (1990–1994), and as a resident, he invented the Airway Cam imaging system to assist in displaying direct laryngoscopy.

Dr. Levitan worked in academic, high-volume, inner-city trauma hospitals in New York City and Philadelphia for 25 years before turning his attention to rural, critical care access hospitals. He now balances clinical duties with teaching courses, speaking engagements, device development, and extensive publishing on laryngoscopy and airway management.

Introduction

Airway management is a critical component of emergency care, and this book is intended to be a refresher on the elements of intubation and the airway.

With this guide, you will learn how to address crisis performance, gain insight on the anatomy of the airway and oxygenation, and brush up on the equipment and processes needed for successful airway management in every patient population. End with an in-depth look at the surgical airway.

Throughout the book, photo sequences offer step-by-step illustrations of an incremental approach to airway management.

Table of Contents

Engineering Crisis Performance

During a crisis, focus on three elements—
cognition, prioritization, and incrementalization—
to maximize your performance.

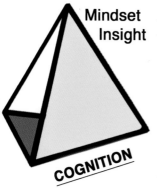

Mindset Insight

Without controlling how you think, you cannot control what you do.

It is the perception of the demand vs. the perception of your abilities that creates performance stress.

If the perceived demands exceed your perceived abilities, your brain triggers an adrenergic response with physiologic and cognitive effects.

Excessive adrenalin causes tachycardia, tremor, altered breathing, muscular tension, lack of situational awareness, loss of visual and auditory cues, and decision paralysis ("stuck on stupid").

Mindset is how you think, how you talk to yourself, and frame the challenges of your job. Managing performance stress, self-talk, and neurolinguistics count.

Procedural insight—true understanding and conviction in a best practice—is required for both confidence and task ownership.

Mindsight coupled with insight lets you accept responsibility, accept reality (be objective), and perform well, even in crisis.

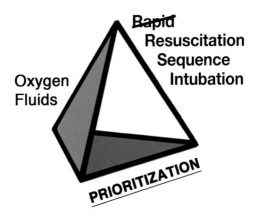

Oxygen
Fluids

~~Rapid~~
Resuscitation
Sequence
Intubation

PRIORITIZATION

In life-and-death human endeavors, crisis performance and survival hinges on proper prioritization.

Complicated algorithms are cognitively crippling and not realistic. Complexity is a fraud. The "big picture" is a distraction; what is required is to focus on and perform the next task.

Oxygenation is the first priority. Hypoxia kills quickly.

Fluids in the airway negate mask ventilation, LMA, apneic oxygenation, and every means of laryngoscopy. Each aspect of management must reduce the risk of regurgitation and emesis and address fluids.

Resuscitate, then intubate, patients in shock. Pharmacologic adjuncts and positive pressure ventilation have hemodynamic consequences. Oxygenation, not plastic, is the urgency in most patients. Ventilation is time-dependent in severe acidosis.

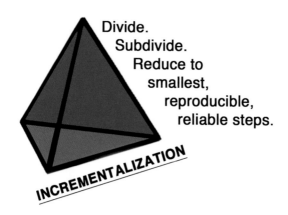

**Divide.
Subdivide.
Reduce to
smallest,
reproducible,
reliable steps.**

INCREMENTALIZATION

The "secret" of competence in crisis is to break down the challenge into smaller parts, and then incrementalize it into its smallest, most fundamental components.

Operators should master a regimented series of best-practice steps that are small, reliable, and reproducible. Expertise is the ability to do each task well, transforming incrementalized steps into one fluid, apparently easy, and effortless movement.

Remember: Slow is smooth, and smooth is fast. Rushing deteriorates performance. Multi-tasking is a myth.

Procedures should be engineered for crisis performance, by flattening the slope and lightening the load.

Slope: Incrementalization
Load: Cognition

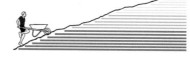

~~Rapid~~ Resuscitation
Sequence Intubation

Rushing has negative effects at multiple points in emergency airway management:

1) Over-ventilation prior to laryngsocopy distends the stomach, increasing the risks of regurgitation and emesis.
2) Jumping the gun on blade insertion, without waiting 60 seconds after RSI meds, can trigger gagging and vomiting.
3) Inserting the blade too quickly, missing the epiglottis on insertion, leads to an inability to recognize landmarks. **It is the most common error of novice intubators.**
4) Inserting the tube too quickly leads to esophageal placement.
5) Over-ventilation post intubation can decrease venous return and trigger hemodynamic collapse.

Optimize pre-oxygenation and apneic oxygenation to prolong safe apnea—allowing for a controlled, calm, slow, and smooth intubation on first pass. Performance improves if you are not rushed by hypoxia. Slow is smooth. Smooth is fast.

Time the laryngsocope insertion to 60 seconds after drugs (closed loop communication with RN). Grip the laryngoscope with 2 fingers, and roll the blade slowly down the curvature of the tongue, with progressive landmark exposure. Insert the tube slowly. Watch the tip enter the glottis.

Optimize oxygenation and fluid status prior to airway management to avoid critical hypoxia and cardiovascular collapse.

Rapid Sequence Intubation should be replaced with the term Resuscitation Sequence Intubation. Resuscitation of critically ill patients should precede intubation.

VAPORS
Airway & Critical Care

Ventilation—Estimate pre-procedural minute ventilation and recognize the extremes of minute ventilation.
Clinical examples: COPD/asthma — low minute ventilation.
Severe acidosis: Compensatory high minute ventilation.

Acidosis—Recognize severe acidosis with compensatory respiratory alkalosis. Examples: severe DKA, salicylate toxicity, acute renal failure, and rhabdomyolysis. In extreme cases it may be difficult to match patient's respiratory effort; therapy treating underlying process may need to be initiated prior to intubation.

Pressures—Note pulmonary pressures and blood pressure. High plateau pressures reduce venous return. Auto-PEEP (breath stacking) can cause hemodynamic collapse. Intubation can cause life-threatening hypotension in critically ill patients.

Oxygenation—Optimize gas diffusion and absorption. Airway strategies must consider alveolar patency, oxygen gradients, safe apnea times, and need for PEEP.

Regurgitation—Overall airway strategy, positioning, and ventilation approaches must prevent emesis and regurgitation, and address handling of fluids. Use an NG tube to decompress bowel obstructions, severe upper GI bleeds, and others at high risk of induction-associated regurgitation.

Shock Index—Heart Rate/Systolic Blood Pressure. Simple ratio for identifying patients at risk of life-threatening hypotension on induction and post-intubation (SI >1.0). Use fluids, titrate induction agents, avoid over-ventilation, and use pressors as needed.

Ventilation

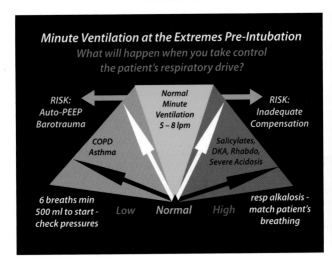

Minute Ventilation at the Extremes Pre-Intubation
What will happen when you take control the patient's respiratory drive?

Normal Minute Ventilation 5 – 8 lpm

RISK:
Auto-PEEP
Barotrauma

RISK:
Inadequate
Compensation

COPD
Asthma

Salicylates, DKA, Rhabdo, Severe Acidosis

6 breaths min
500 ml to start -
check pressures

Low   Normal   High

resp alkalosis -
match patient's
breathing

Ventilatory extremes have much greater risk of peri-intubation clinical deterioration and cardiac arrest.

Minute ventilation = respiratory rate x tidal volume. Normal minute ventilation is 5–8 liters per minute. A respiratory rate of 12 and a tidal volume of 500 = 6 liters minute ventilation. Non-invasive ventilation (CPAP/BiPAP) machines give minute ventilation information directly.

At the extremes of ventilation, general goal (except in apnea) should be to match the patient's own pre-procedure minute ventilation, and then correct ventilatory abnormalities slowly as you treat underlying pathology.

Acidosis & Respiratory Alkalosis

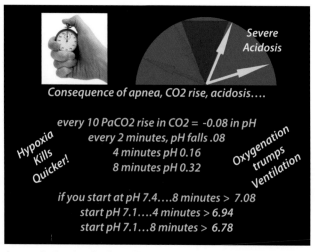

Consequence of apnea, CO2 rise, acidosis....

Severe Acidosis

every 10 PaCO2 rise in CO2 = -0.08 in pH
every 2 minutes, pH falls .08
4 minutes pH 0.16
8 minutes pH 0.32

Hypoxia Kills Quicker!

Oxygenation trumps Ventilation

if you start at pH 7.4....8 minutes > 7.08
start pH 7.1....4 minutes > 6.94
start pH 7.1...8 minutes > 6.78

Apnea during intubation efforts, even of several minutes, is not a problem in most patients, as long as passive oxygenation is effective and hypoxia is avoided.

Patients wth critical hypoxemia despite oxygen (i.e. ARDS, CHF, etc.) and requiring PEEP, fast ventilatory rates, and low tidal volumes—will not tolerate apnea well. CO2 rise is dangerous in patients with increased ICP (cerebral blood flow = MAP-ICP). Increasing PaCO2 leads to an increase in intracerebral pressures.

Apnea (and underventilation) during and after intubation is dangerous in severely acidotic patients with a compensatory respiratory alkalosis. Drop in pH is more precipitous in critically ill than standard formulas above suggests. Below pH of 7.0 there is risk of cardiovascular compromise.

Pressures

Airway Pressures, Blood Pressure and Hemodynamics

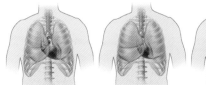

Hyper-inflation after intubation can compress the heart and cause life-threatening hypotension in a COPD patient.

Patients with severe COPD and asthma have a 10x risk of life-threatening peri-intubation hypotension. With excessive rate and volumes the underlying lung pathology prevents air egress. As the lungs expand and pressure rises, auto-PEEP ensues, venous return is compromised, and the heart collapses.

In severe COPD and asthma set the post-intubation ventilation rate to 6 and tidal volume of 500 cc; minute ventilation = 3 lpm. Maximize your inflow rate, allowing maximal time for exhalation between breaths. Correct hypercarbia and increase minute ventilation slowly as you treat underlying disease process. Permissive hypercapnea is well tolerated if pH is kept above 7.0. Aim for plateau pressures <30. Use ketamine drip along with standard therapies if necessary post-intubation.

If pulse oximetry and blood pressure falls post-intubation, slow rate and volume, and check plateau pressures. Disconnect the ventilator, and press on the chest if needed; this will decompress any excess trapped air caused by auto-PEEPing. Verify depth of tube insertion. If tube is in place and disconnecting circuit does not fix the problem, assess for barotrauma and suction the tube.

Oxygenation

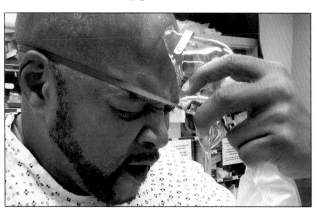

Head forward, upright positioning, and breathing faster are the body's innate responses to hypoxia. Inspiratory flow rates in the trachea exceed the 15 lpm from standard non-rebreather masks.

Patients naturally breathe in through their nose and out their mouth. Face masks create an admixture of exhaled CO_2 and O_2. Providing oxygen via the nose results in a higher FiO_2 in the hypopharynx than face masks at equivalent flow rates.

Patients pull masks off their face because: 1) they provide inadequate flow rates; and 2) they force rebreathing of exhaled CO_2, which effectively lowers the delivered FiO_2.

Adding a nasal cannula to a non-rebreather or CPAP mask augments flow, boosts the effective FiO_2, flushes the naso-pharynx, and generally improves patient tolerance of masks.

Oxygenation

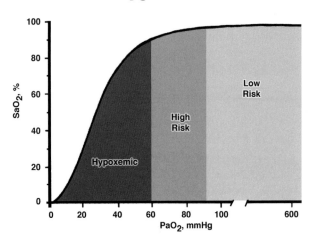

Pulse oximetry is a poor predictor of safe apnea times.

Patients with pulse oximetry readings in the 92-96% range on supplemental oxygen are at high risk of desaturation during intubation. Pulse oximetry in the mid 90s is immediately adjacent to the dropoff point of the pulse oximetry curve.

PEEP and supplemental ventilation (via BVM+cannula or CPAP) should be used on patients who cannot achieve oxygen saturation above 92% with supplemental oxygen.

Nasal **O**xygen **D**uring **E**fforts **S**ecuring **A** **T**ube (**NO DESAT**) provides apneic oxygenation via the nasopharynx during oral intubation, while a laryngoscope blade opens the airway.

Regurgitation

Patients at high risk of regurgitation on induction, those with a distended stomach and small bowel, should have gastric decompression prior to intubation. Examples include the bowel obstructed and upper GI bleeders.

Head elevation (head higher than stomach) helps minimize fluid pooling in hypopharynx and also improves oxygenation if there is fluid in the lungs. Perform laryngoscopy with suction ready.

Time laryngosciopy after muscle relaxants to avoid jumping the gun, i.e., starting too early before full onset of muscle relaxation may trigger gagging (have person giving drugs time 60 seconds).

Shock Index

Shock Index = HR / SBP. Shock Index > 1.0 = high risk of peri-intubation hypotension and cardiovascular collapse.

Patients on negative chronotropic agents or in cardiogenic shock may not elevate their heart rate. Ultrasound is helpful for assessing RV function.

Positive pressure ventilation, loss of adrenic tone, and muscular relaxation can cause hypotension with RSI. Verify good IV function and always fill the tank prior to RSI (fluids, or blood as needed). Initate resuscitation of patients in shock before RSI.

Have push-dose pressors ready, or start IV pressors (usually norepinephrine) prior to intubation with SI > 1.0 after fluids.

Anatomy
Upper Airway

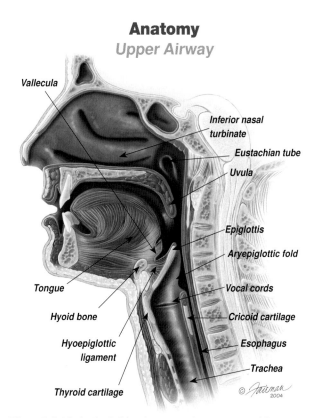

The epiglottis is the bridge between the tongue and larynx.

The esophagus is a flat structure behind the trachea; the larynx is in close proximity to the anterior cervical spine.

The hyoid and hyo-epiglottic ligament suspend the epiglottis from the base of the tongue.

The laryngeal inlet faces posteriorly. Trachea follows the spine.

Anatomy
Upper Airway

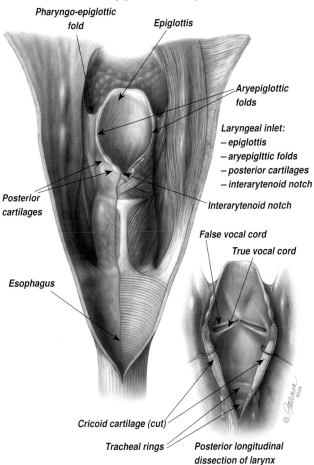

Pharyngo-epiglottic fold

Epiglottis

Aryepiglottic folds

Laryngeal inlet:
– epiglottis
– aryepiglttic folds
– posterior cartilages
– interarytenoid notch

Posterior cartilages

Interarytenoid notch

Esophagus

False vocal cord

True vocal cord

Cricoid cartilage (cut)

Tracheal rings

Posterior longitudinal dissection of larynx

13

Anatomy
Larynx

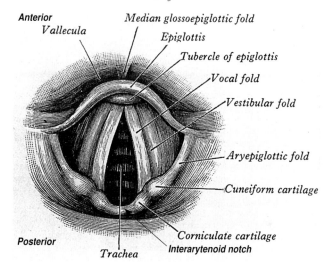

Anterior
Vallecula

Median glossoepiglottic fold

Epiglottis

Tubercle of epiglottis

Vocal fold

Vestibular fold

Aryepiglottic fold

Cuneiform cartilage

Corniculate cartilage

Interarytenoid notch

Posterior

Trachea

The larynx at mirror laryngoscopy, during breathing.

From this perspective the ring of structures making up the laryngeal inlet (epiglottis, aryepiglottic fold, cuneiform and corniculate cartilages, the interarytenoid notch) appear to be on the same plane. This is not the case; the epiglottis is significantly more cranial than the posterior cartilages and notch.

The true vocal cords are caudal to the false cords, and the false cords are caudal to the arytepiglttic folds.

The posterior cartilages, a.k.a., the arytenoids, are located at the top of the cricoid cartilage.

Anatomy
Larynx

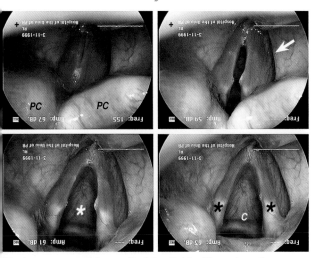

Stroboscopy combines a flashing light with a microphone capturing the vibrations of voice. This allows incredible imaging of the larynx during all phases of phonation and breathing. The vocal cords and posterior cartilages come together during phonation (top left), and open during breathing (bottom right).

Solid white arrowhead is the false vocal cord (top right) , which is just a mucosal fold lateral to and more cephalad than the true vocal cords (black asterisks). PC = posterior cartilages (top left). The epiglottis is marked by a black cross (top images).

The cricothyroid membrane, seen from above, is marked by the black asterisk in lower left image. Note the large cricoid ring, marked C. It is more prominent than the tracheal rings below.

Anatomy
Video Endoscopy

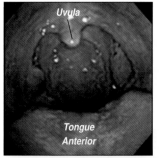

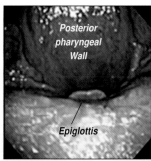

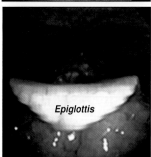

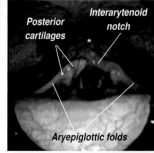

Progressive landmarks during high-resolution endoscopy.
Perspective is facing patient; tongue, epiglottis are below (anterior), posterior cartilages and esophagus above.
"H" marks internal hyoid prominence, "T" the tubercle of the epiglottis, "P" = pyriform.

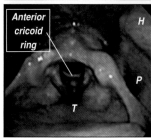

Anatomy
Surgical Exposure in Cadaver

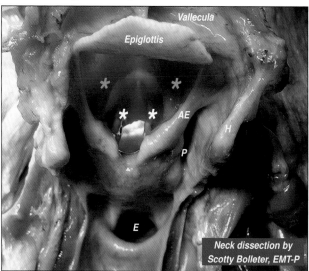

Vallecula

Epiglottis

AE

H

P

E

Neck dissection by Scotty Bolleter, EMT-P

Looking from above at exposed larynx and esophagus after a horizontal surgical incision below the level of the mandible.

The cricothyroid membrane has been incised and is the bright light at center of image seen between the vocal cords.

The true cords are marked with white asterisks, the false cords blue asterisks.

"H" = hyoid (right), which curves in a horseshoe shape around the base of epiglottis, "E" = esophagus. AE = aryepiglottic fold (right). P = pyriform sinus (right). Between the esophagus and interarytenoid notch is the broad, flat back wall of the cricoid. cartilage (unmarked).

Anatomy
Mouth & Neck Mechanics

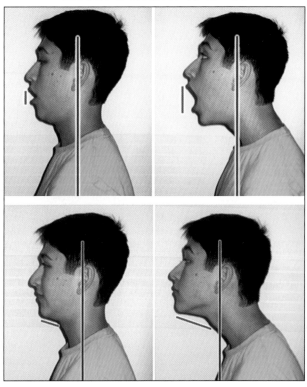

Images on the right show appropriate ear-to-sternal notch position (blue lines), which creates a more anatomically advantageous view of the airway. Images on the left show wider mouth opening and thyromental distance (red lines), allowing greater tongue displacement and straightening the cervical trachea.

Anatomy
Mouth & Neck Mechanics

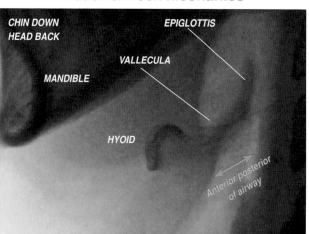

CHIN DOWN
HEAD BACK

EPIGLOTTIS

VALLECULA

MANDIBLE

HYOID

Anterior/posterior of airway

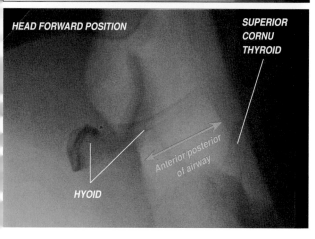

HEAD FORWARD POSITION

SUPERIOR
CORNU
THYROID

Anterior/posterior of airway

HYOID

Anatomy
Mouth & Neck Mechanics

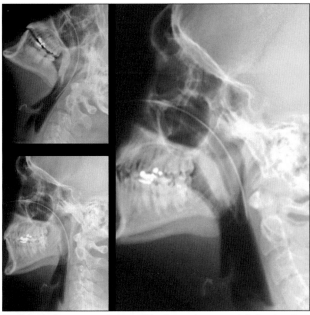

Radiographs comparing positioning: atlanto-occipital extension (top left), chin down and straight head position (bottom left), vs. head forward, ear-to-sternal notch position (right). A tracheal tube is in the nasopharynx and just above the larynx.

Bringing the head forward expands upper airway dimensions, and aligns the upper airway to the cervical and thoracic trachea.

Notice how close laryngeal structures are to the cervical spine; the larynx has mobility side to side, not back.

Anatomy of the Trachea

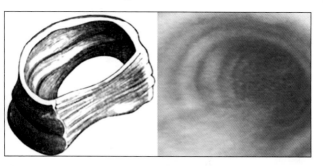

Understanding the anatomy of the trachea is important when addressing tube insertion problems.

The trachea is corrugated (tracheal rings) and has an average diameter of 15–20mm in males and 14–16mm in females.

Tube insertion can be impeded by the tracheal rings and the posterior inclination of the trachea, which follows the thoracic spine. Standard tracheal tubes have an asymmetric left bevel and a leading edge that impacts the anterior tracheal rings.

Stylets add stiffness to the tube and should not be over-bent. They often are shaped with long axis dimensions that exceed the dimensions of the trachea.

The membranous trachea is flat and abuts the esophagus. Objects in the esophagus can cause occlusion if they are pressed into the membranous trachea.

Apneic Oxygenation

Oxygen absorption is dependent on an oxygen gradient, open alveoli, hemoglobin, and forward blood flow. It continues even without movement of the diaphragm, i.e., even during apnea.

Apneic oxygenation has only recently been included in ACLS protocols, but it has a long history in anesthesia, ENT, and thoracic surgery.

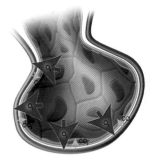

25x more oxygen comes in than CO2 goes out during apnea

Due to the differences in oxygen absorption (250 ml per minute, driven by hemoglobin binding and forward blood flow) and CO2 diffusion (into alveolar space at only 10 ml per minute), there is a negative pressure in the alveolus during apnea. This negative pressure (-240 ml) draws O2 down the trachea during apnea.

CO2 builds up during apnea, at approximately 3–5 mm/Hg per minute. This is rarely consequential during airway management, except in situations of extreme acidosis with compensatory respiratory alkalosis. It can also be consequential in patients with increased intracranial pressure.

Apneic oxygenation does not work well when alveoli are collapsed (i.e., flat positioning in a morbidly obese patient), in ARDS, severe CHF, or other situations when ventilation with PEEP is necessary to stent open the alveoli.

Response to Hypoxia
Patient flat is the coffin position!

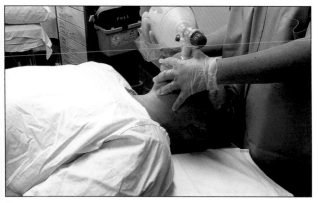

Flat positioning not only increases the risk of regurgitation, but also negatively impacts oxygenation:

1) The tongue and epiglottis fall backwards, creating upper airway occlusion.
2) Dependent alveoli are compressed.
3) Total lung volume is diminished.
4) Diaphragmatic excursion is impacted by abdominal contents
5) The stomach, esophagus, and oropharynx are at the same level, promoting regurgitation of stomach contents as muscular tone is lost.

Mask ventilation is very challenging for a single operator. Even with assistance, pressing the mask down on the face to create a seal pushes the mandible posteriorly—creating obstruction.

Incrementalized Response to Hypoxia
Oxygen On, Pull on the mandible,
Sit the patient up: OOPS

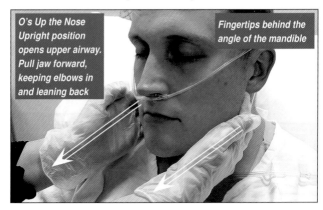

O's Up the Nose Upright position opens upper airway. Pull jaw forward, keeping elbows in and leaning back

Fingertips behind the angle of the mandible

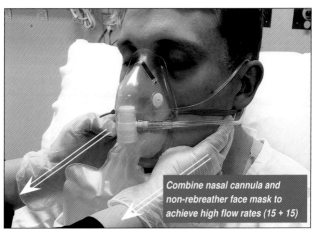

Combine nasal cannula and non-rebreather face mask to achieve high flow rates (15 + 15)

Incrementalized Response to Hypoxia
Bagging upright, with PEEP valve and nasal oxygen under BVM

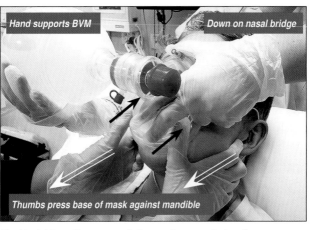

Hand supports BVM • Down on nasal bridge • Thumbs press base of mask against mandible

1) Upright position expands lung volume and alveoli.
2) Upright position allows for diaphragmatic excursion.
3) Upright position lessens risk of passive regurgitation.
4) O's up the nose stents open the airway.
5) O's up the nose provides continuous flow of oxygen even when not squeezing bag (apneic oxygenation).
6) PEEP valve on BVM helps alveolar expansion, O2 absorption.
7) Base of tongue and epiglottis are pulled forward.
8) Seal at base of mask is provided by the operator distracting the mandible. Thumbs press down against mask while fingers pull on mandible—easy mechanism for creating a tight seal, without posterior directed force on mandible (obstructing airway).

O's Up the Nose & the Nasopharynx
The Fire Door of the Airway

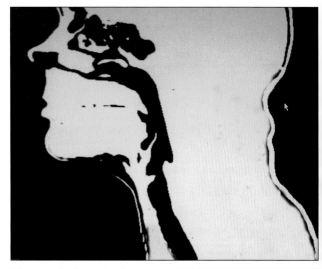

The nose is the natural and better route to oxygenate and to ventilate than the mouth.

Blowing oxygen into the nasopharynx stents opens the airway, which acts like a fire door— it opens as it gets pressurized. The mouth is an an inward opening fire door—it collpases on pressurization.

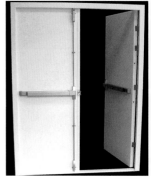

O's Up the Nose & the Nasopharynx
The Fire Door of the Airway

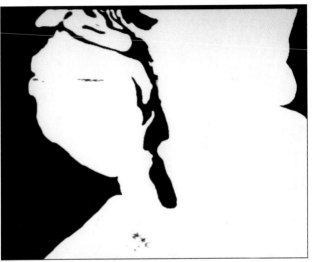

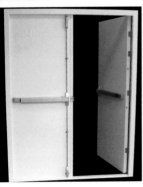

The nasopharynx is the naturally patent airway, even in obese patients.

The nose is a direct and straighter route of gas flow to the trachea.

The nasopharynx is an oxygen reservoir that fills with nasal cannula oxygen during exhalation.

High Flow Nasal Cannula

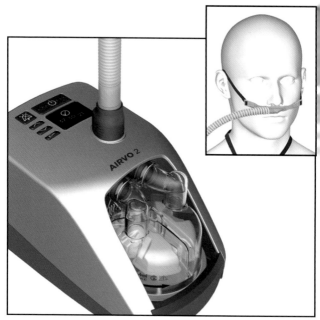

High Flow Nasal Cannula systems combine adjustable flow rates and adjustable FiO2, with humidification. They are much better tolerated than CPAP facemask systems.

High flow rates provide a small measure of PEEP.

Flow rates can be as high as 90 lpm. Rates above 30–40 liters significantly help overcome the work of breathing. Flow rates of 70 lpm have been shown to provide apneic oxygenation and even effective ventilation.

Mask Ventilation in Supine Patient

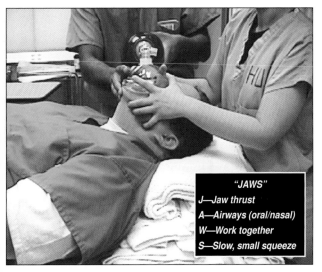

> **"JAWS"**
> J—Jaw thrust
> A—Airways (oral/nasal)
> W—Work together
> S—Slow, small squeeze

Bagging in an ear-to-sternal notch position is better than bagging flat. Bagging upright is best. Tilt the foot of bed down to lower the stomach and improve diaphragmatic excursion. Add nasal cannula and PEEP to all BVM efforts (not shown here).

The operator should use only one hand under the bag, squeezing the bag slowly (1–2 seconds), and using low volume (half the bag) and low rate (6–8 per minute). Cases of compensatory respiratory alkalosis require higher minute ventilation.

A second operator should focus on creating a face mask seal and pulling up on the mandible.

Supraglottic Airways (SGAs)
Redefining Elective Anesthesia and Rescue Ventilation

"Supraglottic airways" refer to airway devices that create an airway seal above the glottis.

LMA type devices have a wedge shaped mask, the tip of which fits behind the cricoid cartilage, in the upper esophagus. The soft tissue above and around the larynx collapses onto the mask. The seal comes from how well the mask mirrors the patient's airway anatomy; it is not a function of how much air is in the mask. Over-inflation causes the mask to be stiffer, worsening the seal and compromising performance. Seal pressure is not related to cuff pressure. LMA devices have lower seal pressures (max ~25 mm Hg) than a tracheal tube or two balloon device.

The Combitube™ and the King LT™ laryngeal tube are supraglottic airways that seal the hypopharynx with one balloon, and the esophagus with a smaller, second balloon. Between the two balloons are ventilation holes, overlying the larynx. Seal pressure with these devices is related to cuff pressure.

SGAs work in 95% of cases of impossible mask ventilation. They work well in supine patients without muscular tone, and also in obesity (unlike mask ventilation).

Muscle relaxants—generally chosen to improve laryngoscopy conditions—also improve mask ventilation and permit SGA insertion without the risk of vomiting. All SGAs require an absent gag response. Over-ventilation through SGAs can cause stomach distention and regurgitation.

Laryngeal Mask Airway

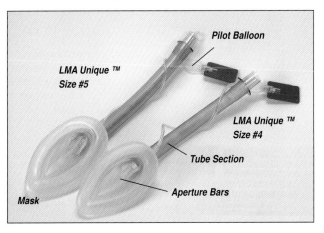

Pilot Balloon

LMA Unique ™ Size #5

LMA Unique ™ Size #4

Tube Section

Aperture Bars

Mask

The Unique™ is the single use version of the original LMA design. It is a "first generation" LMA device. It has a long airway tube, a flat mask, aperture bars, and no gastric decompression port.

The Aintree catheter is a tube introducer that fits over anendoscope that is used to intubate with a standard LMA. It is passed through the LMA into the trachea, the LMA is removed, and then a tube can be railroaded into the trachea.

There are numerous insertion technqiues; for novice and infrequent users, the simplest method is to choose a size 4 for all adult patients, inflate the mask with 15 cc, and insert it around the tongue, aiming it posteriorly on insertion.

Best perfomance happens with half-inflation. The LMA provides rescue ventilation in 95% of mask ventilation failures.

Laryngeal Mask Airway

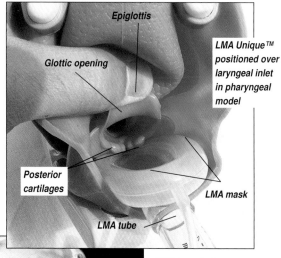

Epiglottis

Glottic opening

LMA Unique™ positioned over laryngeal inlet in pharyngeal model

Posterior cartilages

LMA mask

LMA tube

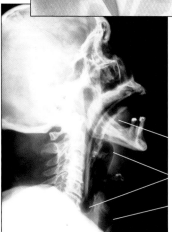

LMA-type devices wedge into the upper esophagus, the mask faces anteriorly, and the larynx collapses backward onto the mask.

LMA tube

LMA mask

Trachea

i-gel LMA-type SGA without a Cuff

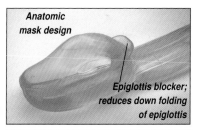

Anatomic mask design

Epiglottis blocker; reduces down folding of epiglottis

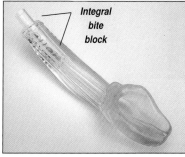

Integral bite block

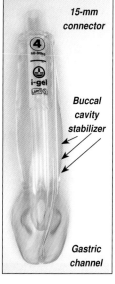

15-mm connector

Buccal cavity stabilizer

Gastric channel

The i-gel has a sophisticated anatomic mask design that does not use a cuff, but instead is made of a thermoplastic elastomer that adapts to the patient's anatomy.

Its broad, flat back helps guide it to proper positioning, and it has more lateral stability than the LMA. It has a gastric decompression channel and comes with a small gastric tube.

Sizes are equivalent to an LMA, i.e., size 4 for most adults, a #5 for large men, and size #3 for very small adults.

air-Q® LMA-type SGA

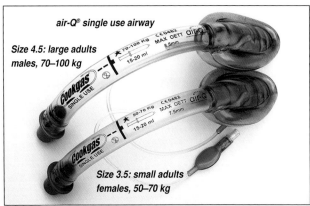

air-Q® single use airway

Size 4.5: large adults
males, 70–100 kg

Size 3.5: small adults
females, 50–70 kg

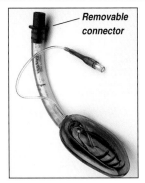

Removable
connector

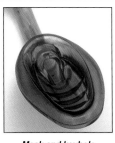

Mask and keyhole
airway outlet

The Cook Gas air-Q® is a second-generation LMA-type device that, like the i-gel, has a sophisticated bowl design, and has the capacity to intubate directly through the device (using an endoscope). It also comes in versions with a self-pressurizing mask or an esophageal block.

AMBU® AuraGain™ LMA-type SGA

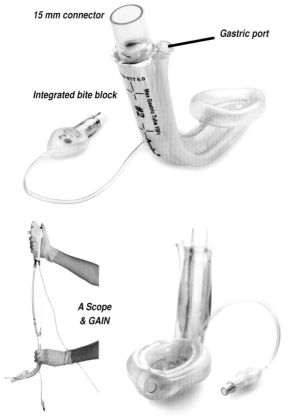

15 mm connector

Gastric port

Integrated bite block

MAX ETT 5.0
Max Gastric Tube 10Fr
#2
Aur...

A Scope & GAIN

The AuraGain™ is an LMA-type SGA designed for endoscopic **intubation** (single-use A scope shown) that also provides gastric decompression.

Endoscopy through the LMA

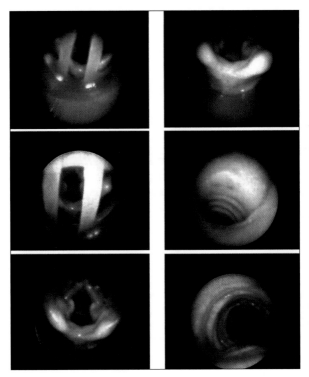

To understand how an LMA-type device fits, it's very useful to see it in situ, through an endoscope. Top left image shows the mask tip (inferior, gray color) going under posterior cartilages, into the upper esophagus. The aperture bars of this LMA Unique™ overlie the larynx. Subsequent images show landmarks as the endoscope moves through the glottis and into the trachea.

Combitube™
2-Balloon Supraglottic Airway

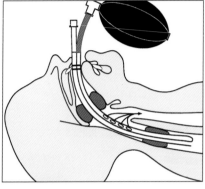

Combitube™ in esophagus. Ventilation through lumen #1 (blue).

Device is available in adult and small adult (SA) sizes. Use SA size for most adults (less than 6.5 ft tall).

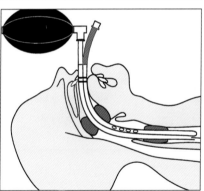

Combitube™ in trachea. Ventilation through lumen #2 (clear).

Be certain to check end tidal CO2 and verify location in all patients so you ventilate through the correct port. Ventilating through the wrong port can be catastrophic.

The Combitube™ is the original 2-balloon device, with 2 lumens and separate ventilation ports. Intended placement is in esophagus (shown top). SA size (small adult) is best for most adults.

King LT™
2-Balloon SGA

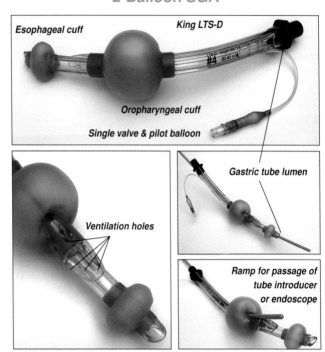

Esophageal cuff

King LTS-D

#4

Oropharyngeal cuff

Single valve & pilot balloon

Ventilation holes

Gastric tube lumen

Ramp for passage of tube introducer or endoscope

The King LT™ has a similar design to Combitube™, but shorter length. The balloons are much softer and share a single inflation port. There is only one ventilation port. This reduces the risk of catastrophic error (ventilating wrong lumen). Insert the device fully, inflate balloons, and then withdraw, veriyfing good ventilation. Recommended to use only the LTS-D version (shown above) with a gastric tube lumen.

Tube Delivery
Direct & Hyperangulated

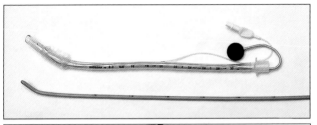

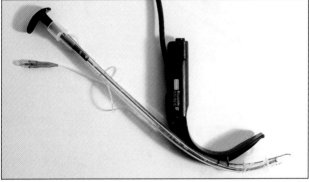

With **conventionally shaped laryngoscope blades** (direct or video), there is a direct line of sight to the target. Insertion is easiest with a straight instrument that has a long, narrow axis. This can be achieved with a straight-to-cuff styletted tube or a bougie (shown in top image).

With a **hyperangulated blade**, a stylet is used to follow the blade around the tongue to reach the target, but this "tongue turner" cannot be passed into the trachea. It exceeds the dimensions of the trachea and is not aligned with tracheal direction.

Tube Delivery Devices
Respecting the Dimensions of the Trachea

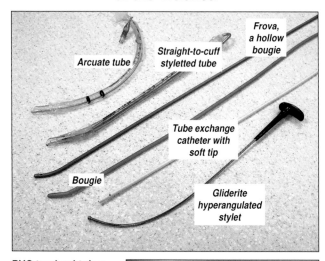

Frova, a hollow bougie

Straight-to-cuff styletted tube

Arcuate tube

Tube exchange catheter with soft tip

Bougie

Gliderite hyperangulated stylet

PVC tracheal tubes have an arcuate shape, making them difficult to insert.

Straight-to-cuff styletted tubes (bend < 35 degrees), and bougies respect the anatomic dimensions of the trachea (15–20 mm in males, 14–16 mm in females).

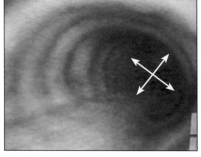

Tube Delivery
Coming from Below Line of Sight

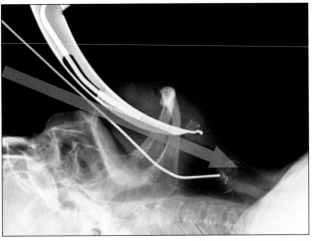

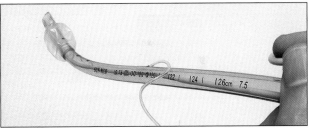

Tracheal tubes must be inserted carefully to avoid moving into the line of sight and blocking the target. Radiograph shows straight-to-cuff styletted tube (below) inserted in the mouth, having been moved toward larynx, now pivoting over posterior structures, and coming from below line of sight to the target.

Tube Insertion
Corrugation & Inclination

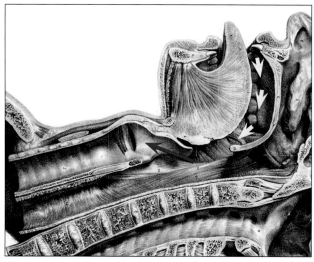

The trachea descends into the thorax, following the thoracic spine. The inclination of the trachea (white) is different than the axis of the laryngeal inlet (pale red) and the curvature around the tongue (yellow).

The anterior tracheal rings create what is essentially a small, corrugated tube.

Any rigid device that is used to get a tube around the tongue cannot be inserted fully into the trachea, due to the trachea's small dimesion, corrugation, and inclination.

Tracheal Tube Tips and Insertion

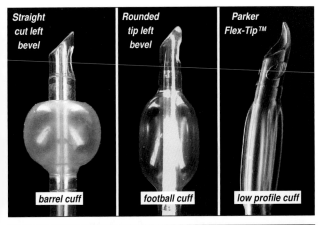

Straight cut left bevel — barrel cuff

Rounded tip left bevel — football cuff

Parker Flex-Tip™ — low profile cuff

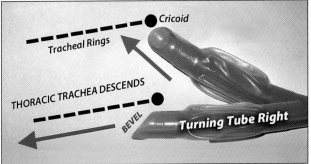

Cricoid

Tracheal Rings

THORACIC TRACHEA DESCENDS

BEVEL

Turning Tube Right

Standard tubes have a left-facing bevel, either with a straight cut, or a slight rounded tip. The Parker Flex-Tip™ tube has a symmetric ski-tip shaped tip. Turning tracheal tubes to the right when they contact the tracheal rings causes the bevel to face upwards and the inclination to turn down, facilitating insertion.

Tube Insertion
with Hyperangulated Stylet

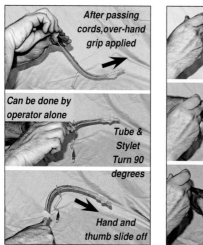

After passing cords, over-hand grip applied

Can be done by operator alone

Tube & Stylet Turn 90 degrees

Hand and thumb slide off

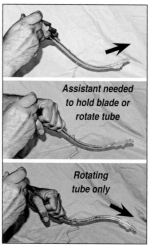

Assistant needed to hold blade or rotate tube

Rotating tube only

The standard approach to dealing with a hyperangulated stylet is to withdraw the stylet after the tube tip is through the cords, and then try pushing the tube down into the trachea. But the tube comes off the stylet pointing upward, following the upward arc of the stylet, not the downward inclination of the trachea (top). This can cause mechanical impaction.

On the left series of images, the stylet and tube are both turned rightward 90 degrees. The tube can then be advanced off the stylet with one hand (can be done without asistance). On the right series, the tube alone is rotated rightward 90 degrees (assistant needed). Either approach solves the problems of corrugation (bevel up) and inclination (tube down).

Tube Introducer
a.k.a. "Bougie"

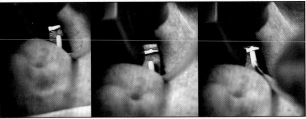

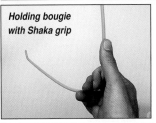

Holding bougie with Shaka grip

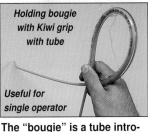

Holding bougie with Kiwi grip with tube

Useful for single operator

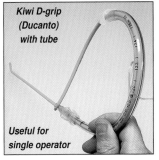

Kiwi D-grip (Ducanto) with tube

Useful for single operator

The "bougie" is a tube introducer with a narrow long-axis and an upturned distal tip.
It has a diameter of 5 mm, smaller than any tracheal tube.

The upturned tip facilitates visualization and bounces off the tracheal rings, providing a tactile confirmation of tracheal placement.

It is useful to know the direction of the upturned tip on placement, especially in poor views. Special grips shown in the photos allow this (unlike a standard pencil grip on the device).

Sliding Tube Over the Bougie into Trachea

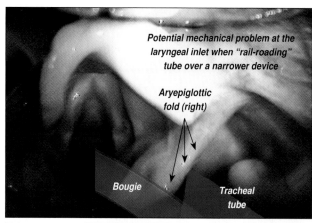

Potential mechanical problem at the laryngeal inlet when "rail-roading" tube over a narrower device

Aryepiglottic fold (right)

Bougie

Tracheal tube

Tubes can catch at the inlet, due to the gap between the outer diameter of the bougie (5mm) or a thin scope, and the ID of a tracheal tube. CCW rotation closes the gap.

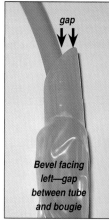

gap

Bevel facing left—gap between tube and bougie

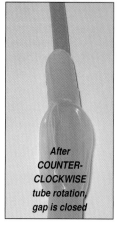

After COUNTER-CLOCKWISE tube rotation, gap is closed

Pre-Intubation Checklist

SOAP–ME;
A mnemonic to prepare for intubation

Suction. Yankauer suction catheter on the right side of the patient's head, within reach of the operator's right hand during laryngoscopy. When properly connected, the suction is audible and palpable when the tip of the catheter is touched against the hand.

Oxygen. Bag valve mask resuscitator with PEEP valve connected to an oxygen source turned all the way up (>15 lpm). The flow of oxygen should be audible and high enough to fill the reservoir bag or tubing. Squeeze bag against hand to verify positive pressure. Nasal cannula on patient.

Airways. Oral and nasal airways and rescue ventilation devices. The cuff of the tracheal tube should be checked and fully deflated. The tracheal tube should be styletted with a straight-to-cuff shape for direct, or hyperangulated at approximately 70 degrees for GlideScope®, Storz D-Blade, or McGARTH® X-blade. Tip of stylet should stop at or before distal edge of cuff, leaving the last 2–3 cm of tube flexible.

Positioning and Pre-Oxygenation. 4 minutes of pre-oxygenation with nasal cannula and mask if possible. Position patient as upright as possible. NC at 4–6 in wide awake, not hypoxic patient; 15 lpm in critically hypoxic, severely dyspneic patient.

Monitoring equipment and Medications. In patients without a pulse, laryngoscopy will occur immediately as monitoring is also being established. With RSI, the patient should have continuous pulse oximetry and cardiac monitoring, and pre-and post-procedure blood pressure monitoring. All medications should be drawn and labeled. The laryngoscopist should clearly communicate with the eam regarding the sequence and timing of medications.

End-tidal CO2 device. All patients require end-tidal CO_2 monitoring, preferably by capnography or capnometry.

Positioning for Intubation

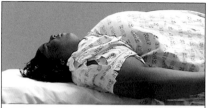

Head elevated laryngoscopy position aligns ear-to-sternal notch.

Multipe benefits for ventilation and laryngoscopy.

Ear-to-sternal notch

In C-spine immobilized patients (and others), tilt the foot of the bed down. This lowers the stomach relative to the mouth and improves pulmonary function.

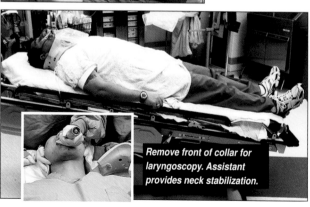

Remove front of collar for laryngoscopy. Assistant provides neck stabilization.

Head Elevation to Improve Laryngoscopy

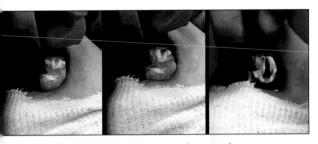

Dynamic lifting of the head improves laryngeal exposure, as shown above. Increasing the head elevation permits greater mouth opening, expands the displacement space, and improves alignment.

While slight head elevation is probably safe in cervical spine immobilized patients, dynamic head elevation is contraindicated if there is a major concern for spine injury.

It is not possible to dynamically lift the obese patient; proper positioning must be done up front. This is best accomplished by using sheets and towels (shown on preceding page) or by using stretch to elevate the head—but you will still need to bring the head forward relative to the chest.

It is best practice to always start laryngoscopy (direct or video) with the patient in ear-to-sternal notch alignment.

Dynamic lifting cannot be done if the patient is positioned too high relative to the operator. The patients' head should be at the position of the operator's belt—not xiphoid, which would prevent any additional head elevation if required.

Pre-Oxygenation & NO DESAT
Nasal Oxygen During Efforts Securing A Tube

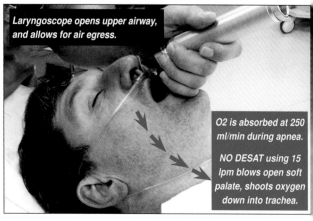

Laryngoscope opens upper airway, and allows for air egress.

O2 is absorbed at 250 ml/min during apnea.

NO DESAT using 15 lpm blows open soft palate, shoots oxygen down into trachea.

Blowing O's up the nose—a.k.a., **NO DESAT**—during laryngoscopy (direct or video) prolongs safe apnea and decreases the incidence of hypoxia during intubation.

NO DESAT can be done with standard nasal cannulas, but does not work well with cannulas designed for CO2 detection, because they have a smaller diameter at the nares (limiting flow).

Use 4–6 liters as part of pre-oxygenation in the wide awake, non-critical patient; 15 lpm if the patient is critically hypoxic. Turn up the flow to 15 lpm on induction. In children—1 lpm/kg.

You need 2 oxygen sources: 1 for BVM (or other mask), and 1 for nasal cannula. If necessary, use a portable tank below the stretcher.

Direct Laryngoscopes
Macintosh & Miller Designs

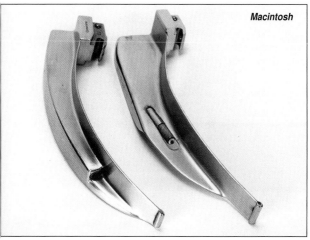

Macintosh

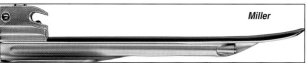

Miller

Conventional direct laryngoscopes come in two major types: curved and straight, though there are many design and performance differences related to method of illumination, dimensions of blade, location of light, etc.

Low flange height designs (i.e., English or German) have many advantages over the Macintosh: a smaller flange that causes less teeth impaction, the ability to use one size in all adults (Mac 4), and better illumination (shorter light-to-tip distance).

Video Laryngoscopes
GlideScope®

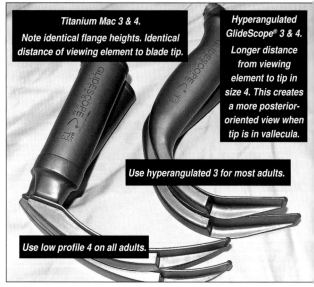

Titanium Mac 3 & 4.
Note identical flange heights. Identical distance of viewing element to blade tip.

Hyperangulated GlideScope® 3 & 4.
Longer distance from viewing element to tip in size 4. This creates a more posterior-oriented view when tip is in vallecula.

Use hyperangulated 3 for most adults.

Use low profile 4 on all adults.

Many manufacturers offer both hyperangulated designs (GlideScope® Titanium standard blades on right) as well as conventional Macintosh designs (GlideScope® Titanium Mac, above left).

Notice that the flange heights on video Mac 3 and 4 are same; the viewing elements are also at the same place relative to the tip. The author advocates a low-profile video Mac for all patients.

Hyperangulated blades have some advantages in patients with severe mobility issues and require less blade insertion than a Mac design, but they often have more difficult tube delivery.

Video Laryngoscopes
Storz C-MAC® System

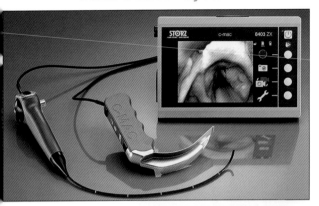

Karl Storz pioneered video laryngoscopes with a conventional Macintosh blade design, the C-MAC®.

An interchangeable video cartridge can fit into a myriad of blades including hyperangulated "D" blade and infant straight blades.

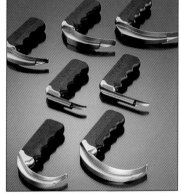

The platform and monitor (top) now also includes endoscopic options, including both short rhinolaryngoscopes (30 cm) and longer intubating bronchoscopes (60 cm).

Video Laryngoscopes
with Integrated Monitors
McGRATH® & King Vision

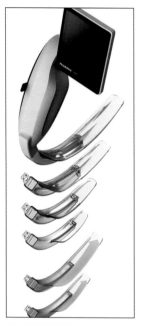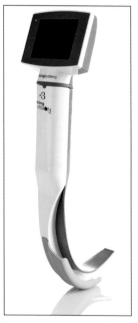

The McGRATH® Mac (left) has both standard geometry Mac blades (2,3,4) and hyperangulated blades (X blade, yellow, 3, 4).

King Vision (right, one size) has an L-bend shape; it comes with and without a channel for tube delivery. The channeled version is shown here. A tube is preloaded into the channel (no stylet) before insertion; it is then slid down the channel into the trachea under video visualization.

Epiglottoscopy
Two-Finger Grip

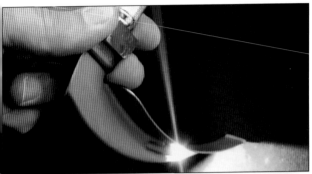

Best practice for direct and video laryngoscopy is largely the same:

1) Epiglottoscopy
2) Progressive landmark exposure
3) Bimanual laryngoscopy (see p. 52); oxygenation, positioning, NO DESAT are identical.

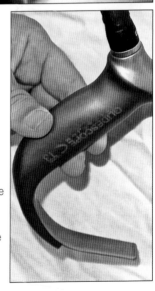

Using a two-finger grip on the laryngoscope, follow the curvature of the blade midline down the tongue; the uvula points to the epiglottis—use light force until the larynx is identified. Use bimanual and head elevation, as needed, for improving the laryngeal view.

Epiglottis
Mechanical & Anatomic Center of the Airway

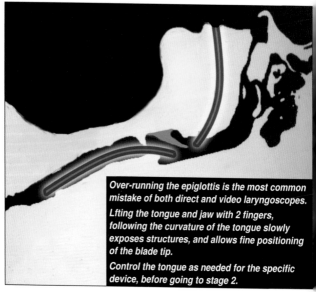

Over-running the epiglottis is the most common mistake of both direct and video laryngoscopes.

Lfting the tongue and jaw with 2 fingers, following the curvature of the tongue slowly exposes structures, and allows fine positioning of the blade tip.

Control the tongue as needed for the specific device, before going to stage 2.

There is only one secret to making laryngoscopy and every intubation a reliable, non-stressful procedure. Find the epiglottis on blade insertion, whether with direct or video laryngoscopes.

The epiglottis is the **mechanical center** of the airway, between the curve of the tongue and the curve of the cervical trachea.

The epiglottis is the **anatomic center** of the airway, connecting the tongue (where we start) to the top of the larynx, our goal.

Epiglottis Camouflage

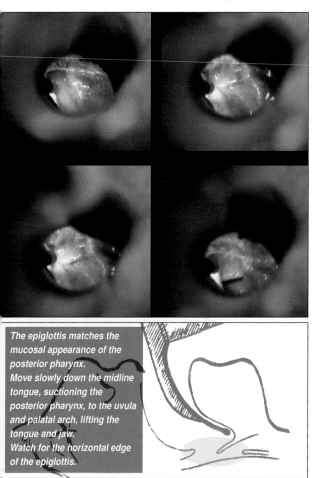

The epiglottis matches the mucosal appearance of the posterior pharynx.
Move slowly down the midline tongue, suctioning the posterior pharynx, to the uvula and palatal arch, lifting the tongue and jaw.
Watch for the horizontal edge of the epiglottis.

Controlling the Tongue
Conventional Blades the Right Corner—
The Pivot Area of Mouth

Tongue control is important for optimizing larngeal exposure, but it is also critical for tube delivery. Here is ideal positioning of the tongue with a curved blade.

The right corner of the mouth is the tube delivery area in direct laryngoscopy.

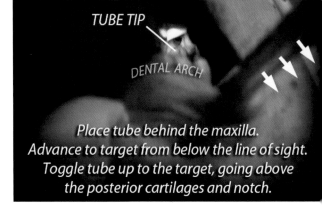

TUBE TIP

DENTAL ARCH

Place tube behind the maxilla.
Advance to target from below the line of sight.
Toggle tube up to the target, going above
the posterior cartilages and notch.

Hyperangulated Blades
Tongue Control, Tube Delivery, and Preventing Injury on Tube Insertion

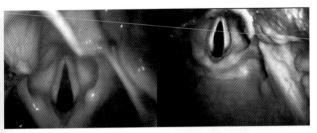

Conventionally shaped video laryngoscope blades (GlideScope® Titanium Mac, Storz C-MAC®, and McGRATH® Mac) are positioned identically to direct laryngoscopy. Start with a midline approach and a light touch to find the epiglottis, then after epiglottoscopy, move to control the tongue, by gently moving blade to the right, and sweeping the tongue to the left side of the mouth. This frees the right corner of the mouth for tube delivery, which is the only place possible to pivot a narrow, straight-to-cuff stylet/tube.

Hyperangulated blades (GlideScope®, Storz D-blade, McGATH® X blade, King Vision) are introduced the same way—with a midline approach coming down the tongue and a light, 2-finger grip. After the larynx is found, however, hyperangulated blades stay midline. Tube delivery follows the blade down to the larynx.

Ideal positioning of a hyperangulated blade has the larynx in alignment with the blade axis, and the larynx at the top half of the video monitor. This permits visualization of the styletted tube as it follows the blade down, in the lower part of the screen. Inserting a styletted tube blindly (off screen) can cause injury.

Stage 2 Grip of Laryngoscope
The Blade as an Extension of the Forearm

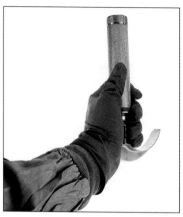

After epiglottoscopy, and the tongue has been controlled, the next step in laryngoscopy is optimizing laryngeal exposure. This requires more force than the first stage of the procedure.

Switch from a 2-finger grip to gripping the handle where it meets the blade. Point your thumb up the handle.

A low grip and thumb up positioning permits fine control.

The blade should be an extension of your forearm.

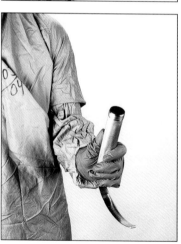

Keep your elbow close to your torso, and lean in to transmit force down the blade, with minimal use of your deltoid.

Bimanual Laryngoscopy
Integral to Development of Laryngoscopy

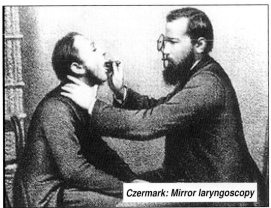

Czermark: Mirror laryngoscopy

The mobility of the larynx and the use of two hands to optimize laryngeal exposure have always been integral to laryngoscopy—whether with a mirror, direct laryngoscope, or now with video laryngoscopes. Bimanual laryngoscopy can move the larynx posteriorly into the line of site and has dramatic effects on indirect epiglottis elevation.

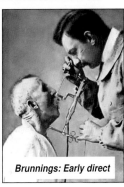

Brunnings: Early direct

As shown in these images, and true with direct laryngoscopy today, the larynx is sighted monocularly. Operators should have visual acuity testing and know which eye they use to site the larynx.

Bimanual Laryngoscopy

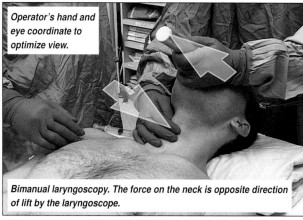

Operator's hand and eye coordinate to optimize view.

Bimanual laryngoscopy. The force on the neck is opposite direction of lift by the laryngoscope.

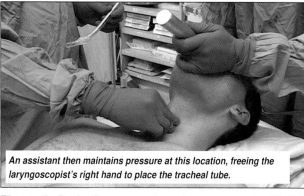

An assistant then maintains pressure at this location, freeing the laryngoscopist's right hand to place the tracheal tube.

Bimanual—By the Operator. Not cricoid pressure and not BURP (Backward Upward Rightward Pressure)—these are done by assistants and do not work as well to optimize exposure.

Bimanual Laryngoscopy
Mechanics

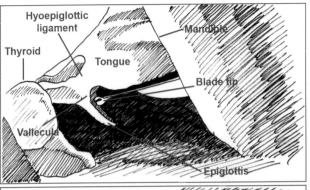

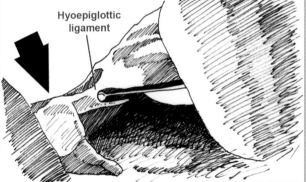

Laryngeal exposure with a curved blade—whether by direct or video—is about subtle mechanical force applied at the base of the epiglottis. The blade tip must be properly placed in the vallecula; bimanual "locks" the tip into the proper position, lifting the epiglottis. It also lowers the larynx into the line of sight.

Bimanual Laryngoscopy and Laryngeal View

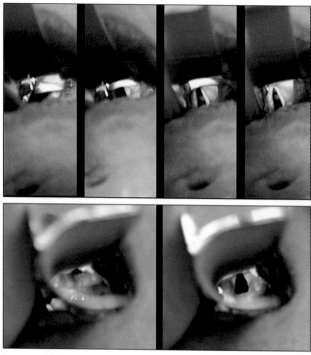

In **curved blades** (top example), bimanual laryngoscopy improves how the blade tip fits into the vallecula, improving indirect epiglottis elevation. The larynx is also lowered into the line of sight.

In **straight blades** (below) the epiglottis has been picked up directly by the tip of the blade. Improvement in laryngeal view is from pushing the larynx downward into the line of sight.

Bimanual Laryngoscopy and Laryngeal View

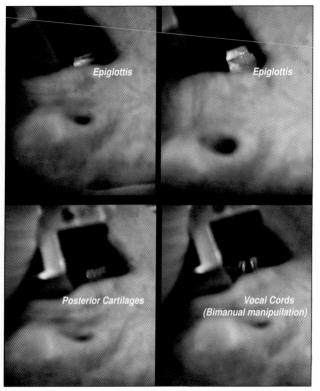

Bimanual laryngoscopy in an elderly woman with no teeth, using a Macintosh blade.

Laryngeal exposure improves dramatically, and a view of only the posterior cartilages is transformed to a view of the cords.

Straight Blade
Lifting Epigottis Directly

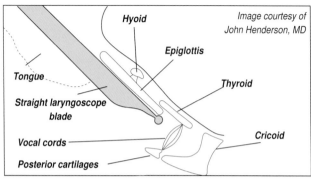

Image courtesy of John Henderson, MD

Hyoid

Epiglottis

Tongue

Thyroid

Straight laryngoscope blade

Vocal cords

Cricoid

Posterior cartilages

Most modern laryngoscopy—with direct or video devices—is done using curved blades and involves indirect epiglottis elevation. Straight blades can be very useful in situations when indirect elevation of the epiglottis is problematic or impossible. This occurs commonly with peri-laryngeal pathology, such as epiglottitis, epiglottic cysts, tumors, polyps, angioedema, etc.

Straight blades are also very useful when the thyromental distance, i.e., the displacement space between chin and thyroid cartilage, is very short. This is the rule in infants and small children, and with an omega-shaped, relatively long epiglottis, indirect control can be difficult.

Straight blades are introduced as curved blades, but then should be moved to the right corner of the mouth (as this is the pivot area where the dental arch arcs backward). The blade tip enters the laryngeal inlet, lifting the epiglottis directly. Tube delivery should be from the extreme right corner of the mouth.

Incrementalized Direct Laryngoscopy
Epiglottoscopy → Laryngoscopy →
Tube Delivery

T -5 minutes: Pre-oxygenation (upright as much as possible) and NG decompression if needed. Verify functioning IV lines.

T -1 minute: RSI — Give induction agent and muscle relaxant, one after the other. RN times and calls out 60 seconds after pushing meds (i.e., when it is safe to attempt blade insertion).

T -1 to Time zero: Increase NC to 15 lpm if not done already (NO DESAT). Gently ventilate with PEEP awaiting muscle relaxation, upright or in ear-to-sternal notch position. Use low rate, volume, and pressure (6–8 ml/kg, 8–12 breaths/min) unless severe acidosis with compensatory respiratory alkalosis.

Time zero: 2-finger grip and light force—for epiglottoscopy and tongue control. Follow curve of blade down tongue midline. Suction posterior pharynx as necessary—expose progressive landmarks: uvula, epiglottis, and larynx. After localizing larynx, control tongue (blade moves right, tongue left). Change to high force grip. Use bimanual laryngoscopy and/or head elevation to augment laryngeal exposure.

Tube delivery is from the right side of the mouth, with straight-to-cuff narrow long-axis stylet shape. Visualize tip passing over notch. If mechanical problem of insertion (catching on tracheal rings) turn tube right. Use bougie as needed.

Verify tube placement with end-tidal CO_2, oximetry, CXR.

Direct Laryngoscopy
Sequence 1: Macintosh Blade & Bimanual

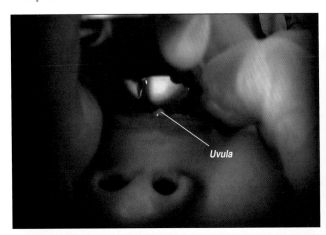

Uvula

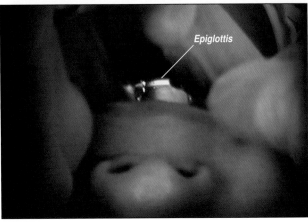

Epiglottis

Direct Laryngoscopy
Sequence 1: Macintosh Blade & Bimanual

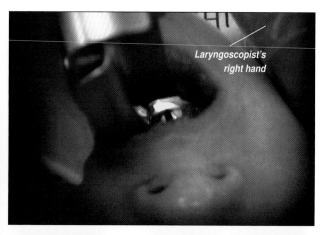

Laryngoscopist's
right hand

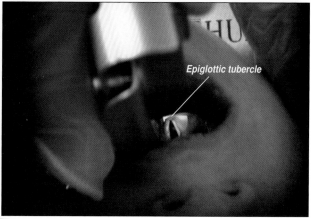

Epiglottic tubercle

Direct Laryngoscopy
Sequence 2: Macintosh Blade

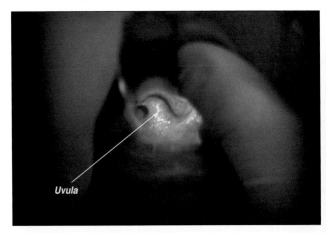

Uvula

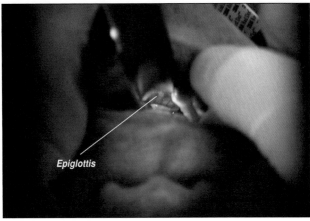

Epiglottis

Direct Laryngoscopy
Sequence 2: Macintosh Blade

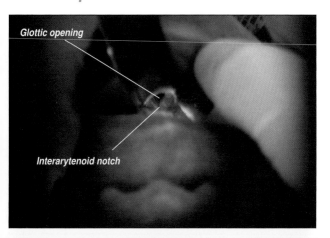

Glottic opening

Interarytenoid notch

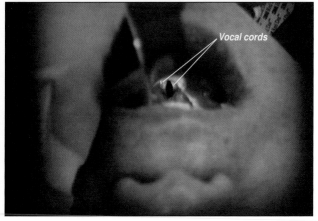

Vocal cords

Direct Laryngoscopy
Sequence 3: Macintosh Blade, Posterior Structures Only

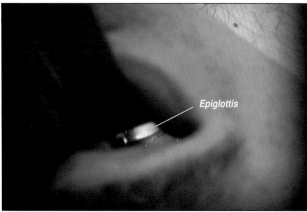

Epiglottis

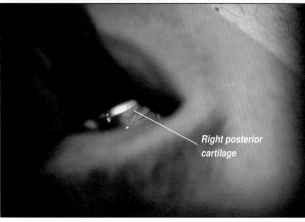

Right posterior cartilage

Direct Laryngoscopy
Sequence 3: Macintosh Blade, Posterior Structures Only

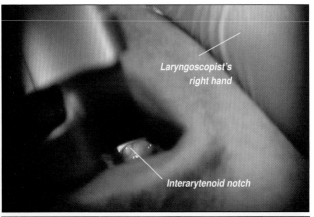

Laryngoscopist's right hand

Interarytenoid notch

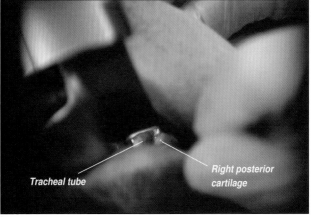

Tracheal tube

Right posterior cartilage

Direct Laryngoscopy
Sequence 4: Straight Blade (Wisconsin)

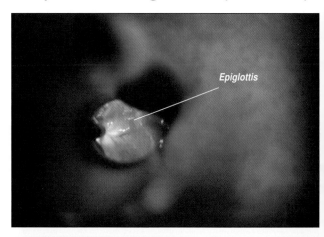

Epiglottis

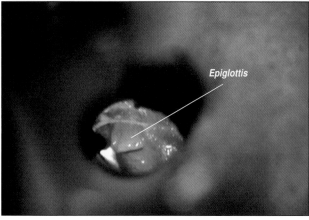

Epiglottis

Direct Laryngoscopy
Sequence 4: Straight Blade (Wisconsin)

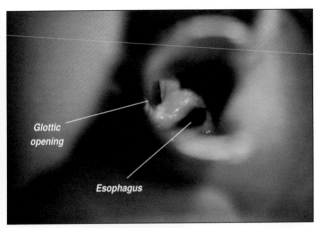

Glottic opening

Esophagus

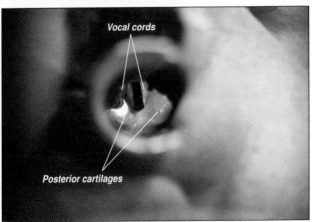

Vocal cords

Posterior cartilages

Problem-Solving
Direct Laryngoscopy

The most common "problem" with direct laryngoscopy is laryngeal exposure. Tube delivery is generally straightforward.

"Difficult" laryngoscopy is commonly overcome by a more experienced operator using the same instrument, i.e., the problem is often the operator, not the device.

Expert laryngoscopists move slowly down the tongue and identify the epigottis on insertion; novices frequently over-run the epiglottis and fail to identify any structures.

Problem: No landmarks seen:
a) Using a 2-finger grip on laryngoscope roll midline down the tongue until epiglottis is identified (uvula points to epiglottis).
b) Dab posterior pharyngeal wall with Yankauer suction tip to discriminate edge of epiglottis as necessary.

Problem: Laryngeal exposure, i.e. epiglottis only view:
a) With light force, adjust tip of blade to fit fully into the vallecula.
b) Apply bimanual laryngoscopy.
c) Increase head elevation (avoid atlanto-occipital extension).
d) If epiglottis is still a problem, use the tip of the curved blade (or straight blade) to lift the epiglottis directly.

Problem: Tube delivery (straight-to-cuff 35 degree bend tube)
a) If resistance is felt on insertion, rotate left-bevel tube/stylet to right, or use bougie.
b) Advance tube from below line of sight, pivot in the right corner of the mouth, and watch tip pass over interarytenoid notch.

Incrementalized
Video Laryngoscopy

Same overall strategy as direct laryngoscopy: epiglottoscopy, laryngoscopy, and tube delivery.

Same pre-oxygenation, positioning, drug timing, nasal cannula (NO DESAT), etc. as direct laryngoscopy.

Time zero: 2-finger grip—epiglottoscopy and tongue control—all with low force. Follow the curve of blade down the tongue midline. The uvula points to the epiglottis. Suction the pharynx as necessary. Same as direct laryngoscopy.

Hyperangulated blades stay midline; conventionally shaped Mac video laryngoscopes control tongue left (blade moves right).

Improve laryngeal exposure with bimanual laryngoscopy or head elevation.

Tube delivery with video devices follows the blade down to the glottis. Directly observe tube insertion in the mouth, move down the blade, and then watch on video as the tube tip enters glottis.

Hyperangulated stylets are used for tube delivery with hyperangulated blades, but cannot be inserted into the trachea. Conventionally shaped video laryngoscope blades use a conventionally shaped stylet/tube (i.e. straight-to-cuff). For channeled video devices, no stylet is used. Adjust the device position as necessary to modify the direction of tube movement from the channel.

Verify tube placement with end-tidal CO_2, oximetry, CXR.

Video Laryngoscopy
Sequence 1

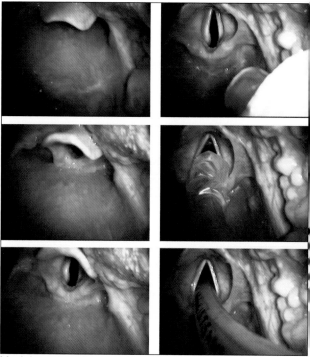

Ideal demonstration of hyperangulated GlideScope® technique.

Low insertion, epiglottoscopy, target is kept in upper half of screen, and laryngeal inlet is aligned with axis of blade.

Tube insertion is visible from the bottom half of the screen, and the tube is clearly seen entering the larynx.

Images courtesy of Richard Cooper, MD

Video Laryngoscopy
Sequence 2

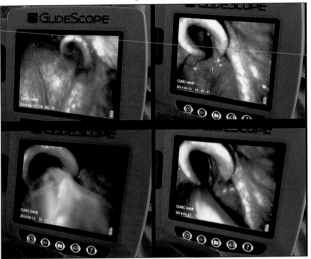

Video laryngoscopy using GlideScope® Titanium Macintosh blade in super-obese man who happens to have a long tubular epiglottis. Initially it was very tough to identify any structures, but epiglottis edge was recognized, and then the blade tip positioned further down the tongue, into the vallecula, using bimanual laryngoscopy.

The cords and glottis are shadowed by the long tubular epiglottis, but the posterior cartilages are seen in top right image.

Tube delivery is done carefully, as the cuff of the tracheal tube transiently blocks the line of imaging (bottom left).

Video Laryngoscopy
Sequence 3

Intubation in a 5-year-old with a Storz C-MAC® video laryngoscope.

Images courtesy of Paul Baker, MD

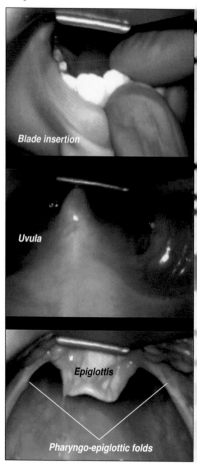

Blade insertion

Uvula

Epiglottis

Pharyngo-epiglottic folds

Video Laryngoscopy
Sequence 3

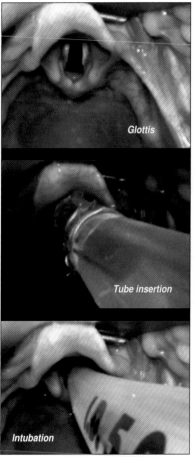

Glottis

Tube insertion

Intubation

After a terrific view of the larynx is obtained, notice that tube insertion causes a transient blockage of the target as the tube moves between the viewing element on the blade and the larynx.

It is important to always verify the tube position after insertion, as shown in the bottom image. The tube is clearly passing above the posterior cartilages and notch.

Tube delivery should always be slow and smooth, avoiding esophageal placement, and also so it is accomplished on first attempt.

Video Laryngoscopy
Sequence 4

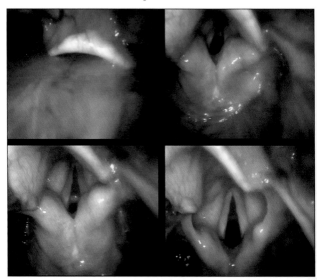

Sequential GlideScope® images in which the hyperangulated blade is over-inserted and off axis relative to the larynx.

The blade has been advanced too far (bottom left), the viewing element is too close to the target, filling screen, and steepening the angle of approach. The epiglottis is pointing leftward because the blade has been positioned right of midline.

Tube insertion is being attempted in the bottom right image, but cannot be seen. This can easily lead to injuries of the palate and tonsils.

Images courtesy of Marvin Wayne, MD

Video Laryngoscopy
Sequence 5

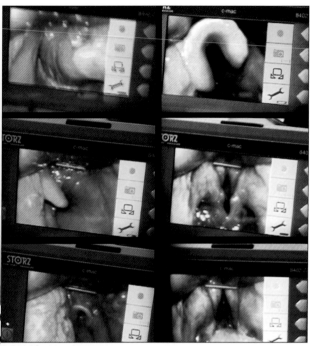

C-MAC® video laryngoscopy in a super-obese man with difficult anatomy. Initial image of generous soft tissue, including the tongue, soft palate, and pharyngo-epiglottic folds. The epiglottis is identified in second image on left, but the large tongue made it dificult to find, and it is way off midline. The next challenge was controlling the epiglottis to achieve exposure and tube delivery. After various attempts at indirect elevation, laryngoscopy and intubation was only possible by lifting tubular epiglottis directly.

Hyperangulated
Video Laryngoscopy
The Angle of Approach

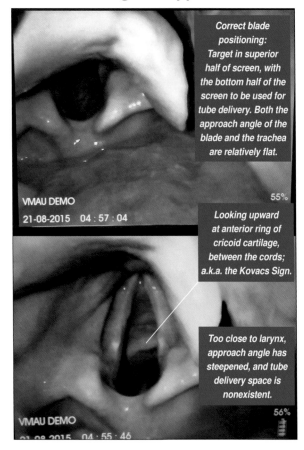

Correct blade positioning: Target in superior half of screen, with the bottom half of the screen to be used for tube delivery. Both the approach angle of the blade and the trachea are relatively flat.

Looking upward at anterior ring of cricoid cartilage, between the cords; a.k.a. the Kovacs Sign.

Too close to larynx, approach angle has steepened, and tube delivery space is nonexistent.

Hyperangulated
Video Laryngoscopy
The Angle of Approach

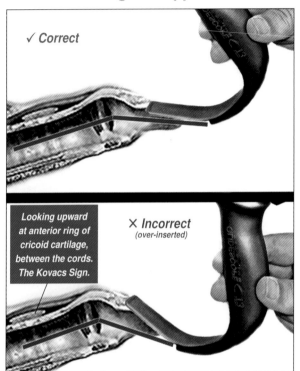

✓ *Correct*

Looking upward at anterior ring of cricoid cartilage, between the cords. The Kovacs Sign.

✗ *Incorrect*
(over-inserted)

Schematic representation of images on opposite page.
Angle of approach is steeper in bottom image, and viewing element is closer to target. Tube insertion has to overcome a more acute angle.

Problem-Solving
Video Laryngoscopy

No landmarks: Back up, and incrementally advance down the center of the tongue, going very slowly, progressively visualizing uvula and palatal arch, dabbing posterior pharyngeal wall with Yankauer. Uvula points to the epiglottis.

No landmarks with hyperangulated blade: Use a smaller blade. The viewing element of a hyperangulated GlideScope® 4 blade comes off farther from the tip of the blade than the hyperangulated GlideScope® 3. For most adults the GlideScope® size 3 is the best choice. Smaller blades also create a less acute angle of approach and often create easier tube delivery.

Difficulty getting tube to target: Use the blade as the conduit to move to larynx. Directly visualize insertion into the mouth, gently advance down the blade until it comes into view on the monitor.

Poor visualization of tube insertion into the larynx: Video laryngoscopes usually provide much better visualization of the tube insertion compared to direct laryngoscopy; however, as the tube moves down the blade, the tube and cuff can obscure the video imaging element. Often it is hard to see the leading edge of a left bevel tube. Manipulate the tube below the video imaging element so you can see the tip coming over the interarytenoid notch.

Difficult tube insertion into trachea: Do not attempt to insert hyperangulated stylet and tube into trachea without addressing corrugation and inclination issues.

Pediatric Intubation Overview

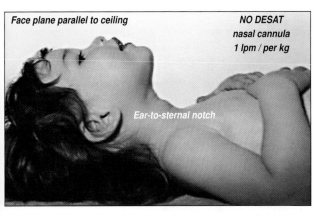

Face plane parallel to ceiling

NO DESAT
nasal cannula
1 lpm / per kg

Ear-to-sternal notch

Pediatric intubation is technically easier than adult intubation.
Poor laryngeal views are 10x less common in children than in adults. The procedure is more stressful to clinicians, making an incrementalized, step-wise approach even more important.

Epiglottoscopy is critical—in infants the uvula and epiglottis touch. The epiglottis is relatively long and can be difficult to control. Infants and children have a short thyromental distance, meaning a small displacement space for the tongue. All of these variables favor the use of straight blades in small children. Straight blades are recommended for infants and most children below the age of 4. Curved blades do better for suctioning in high-volume fluid situations.

Surgical airways in small children require tracheotomy; below the age of 8 cricothyrotomy is not feasible. Infants have more tracheal rings (~10) above the sternal notch vs. adults (4–6).

Pediatric Laryngoscopy
Sequence 1

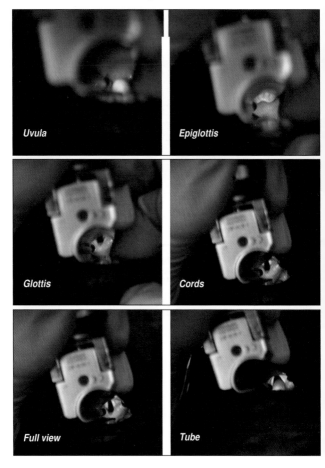

Pediatric Laryngoscopy

Sequence 2

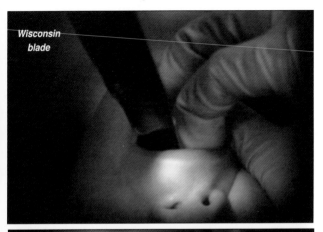

Wisconsin blade

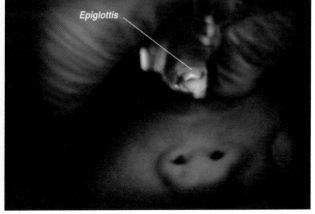

Epiglottis

Pediatric Laryngoscopy
Sequence 2

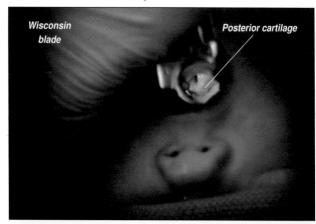

Wisconsin blade

Posterior cartilage

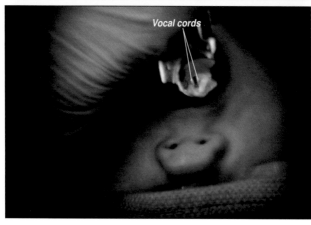

Vocal cords

Pediatric Laryngoscopy
Sequence 3

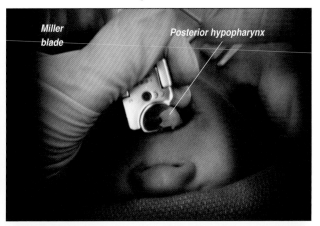

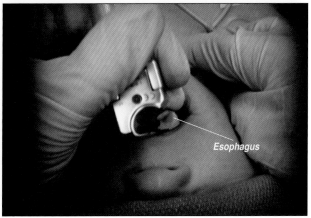

Pediatric Laryngoscopy
Sequence 3

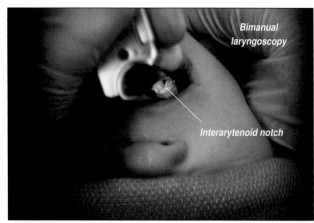

Bimanual laryngoscopy

Interarytenoid notch

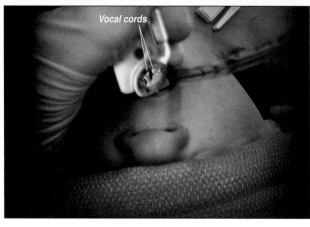

Vocal cords

Pediatric Laryngoscopy
Sequence 4

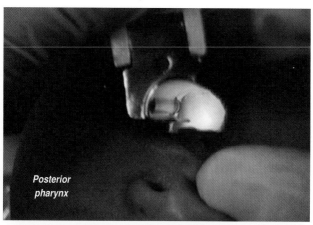

Posterior pharynx

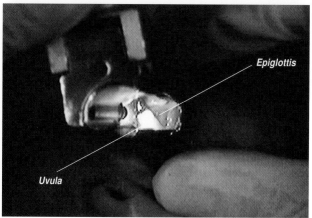

Epiglottis

Uvula

Pediatric Laryngoscopy
Sequence 4

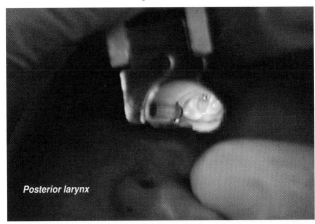

Posterior larynx

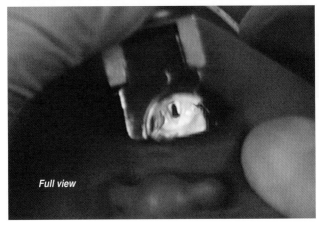

Full view

Decision-Making
Use of Muscle Relaxants

Muscle relaxation (RSI) creates optimal conditions for laryngoscopy oral intubation, insertion of supraglottic airways, and mask ventilation. It also eliminates the risk of active vomiting or gagging, a signifcant risk in emergency airways.

Safety with RSI depends on a redundancy of means to intubate and oxygenate. Oxygenation methods include passive oxygenation, face mask, and supraglottic airways. Video laryngoscopy has significantly increased the margin of safety in intubation. Likewise, supraglottic airways and apneic oxygenation have significantly increased the margin of safety in oxygenation. Tolerance of apnea and the hemodynamic impact of drugs and intubation must also be considered.

In most emergency situations, the benefits of muscle relaxants outweigh the small risks of the "cannot intubate/cannot oxygenate" situation. Intubation without muscle relaxants has its own risks, such as suboptimal conditions, increased likelihood of repeat and prolonged attempts, and vomiting. Additonally, without an absent gag, supraglottic airways cannot be inserted.

RSI is generally avoided when rescue oxygenation and ventilation will not likely work. In such situations, if intubation fails, a surgical airway is required. Time to ventilation with a surgical airway averages 100 seconds. Occasionally muscle relaxants are used in high-risk situations, with concurrent preparations for a surgical airway, i.e. a double set-up. After drug administration, one attempt is made at intubation; a surgical airway is initiated immediately if there is any delay.

Non-RSI Oral Intubation

"Awake" intubation refers to approaches in which patients keep breathing. This can mean different things: 1) topicalization only; 2) topicalization plus some adjunctive sedative agent; 3) topicalization and a large dose of a sedative—which may cause apnea and create significant or even full relaxation in some patients.

The challenge of "awake" oral intubation is predicting patients' response to the stimulus of laryngoscopy, their risk of gagging and vomiting, and their reponse to sedative agents. Certain clinical situations may allow intubation with minimal pharmacologic adjuncts (decreased patient responsiveness, muscular fatigue): hypercarbia, encephalopathy, overdose, sepsis, profound shock, neuromuscular disease, etc. In neonates and infants it is usually easy to physically overcome resistance to laryngoscopy.

When response to laryngoscopy is expected to be minimal, a laryngoscope can be inserted to gauge patient response—and then perform intubation if feasible, or deciding to switch to RSI after assessing the likelihood of intubation success.

Ketamine has unique properties relative to other induction agents and is often chosen for "awake," non-RSI approaches (through mouth, nose, or neck). It is a unique dissociative agent that generally does not impair respiration but creates "cooperation in a vial." Ketamine, combined with topicalization of the airway, gentle insertion of a video laryngoscope, and a bougie is often effective for "awake" oral intubation.

In any "awake"approach, be ready to use RSI medications, manage regurgitation, and adapt to the patient's response.

Non-RSI Nasal Intubation

The nasal route of intubation is chosen in situations of obvious pathology about the mouth and base of tongue.

Nasal intubation can be done with sedatives and muscle relaxation (using a mask system and bronchoscope swivel adapter to provide continuous ventilation during endoscopy, but it is most often chosen because of an expected challenging airway and a desire to keep the patient upright and breathing spontaneously.

Sedation and pharmacologic adjuncts required are less than is necessary for going through the mouth, but vasoconstriction of the nose and topicalization of the nasopharynx and larynx are critical. Ketamine can be used in small aliquots to aid in minimizing movement and patient resistance.

Because a nasal approach is often chosen in situations of obvious anatomic problems with the mouth, operators must anticipate the need for a surgical airway if nasal intubation fails, as many of these patients cannot be effectively oxygenated using mask ventilation or supraglottic airways. Mark the neck and have the surgical airway equipment at bedside.

Blind nasal intubation is feasible, but endoscopic guidance is very helpful and often part of the reason a nasal intubation is being chosen (eg, to inspect the larynx and airway in burns, angioedema, pathology about the tongue, etc.).

There are two basic approaches: 1) Tube first—Tracheal tube is placed in nares to a depth of 12–14cm, then followed by a scope; 2) Tube on scope—The tube is loaded on a scope that is passed from nose to carina, then the tube is railroaded down.

Nasoendoscopy Landmarks

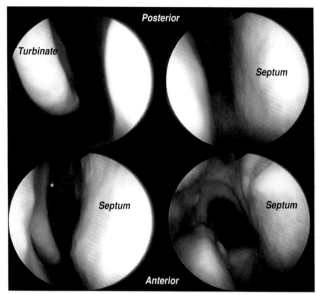

Nasoendoscopy is a valuable tool for airway assessment and is relatively easy to perform. It is especially useful managing and assessing angioedema, burns, vocal cord function, and foreign bodies. Endoscopy is also useful for checking tracheostomies.

Before nasoendoscopy, spray the nares with topical anesthetic and vasoconstrictant. Have nothing behind the patient's head.

The basic "rules" of endoscopy are:
- Know your starting position and proceed slowly.
- Maintain a perspective on critical landmarks.
- Follow the open channel.

Nasoendoscopy Landmarks

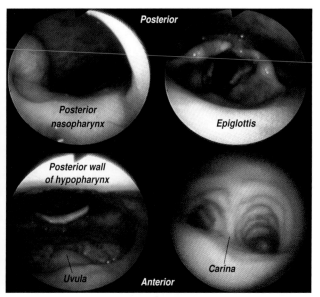

Visually insert the scope in open nares. Be gentle in the first 1 inch, navigating around the inferior turbinate and any septal spur. When you reach the back of the nasopharynx, have the patient breathe through the nose and lean slightly forward.

The scope is passed back through the nasopharynx, then downward over the posterior nasopharynx to the hypopharynx, where the epigottis and larynx should come into view. Try to avoid touching the posterior pharyngeal wall and epiglottis.

The bottom right image shows a view of the carina (seen with 60 cm bronchoscope, not 30 cm rhinolaryngoscope).

Nasal Intubation
Specialized Equipment

Trigger tubes allow flexion of the distal tip of the tube by pulling on the ring.

Endotrol® has a left bevel, so a counterclockwise rotation is needed as the tube is slid off the scope; this is not needed with the Parker tip.

The trumpet should always precede the tube.

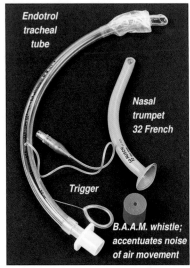

Endotrol tracheal tube

Nasal trumpet 32 French

Trigger

B.A.A.M. whistle; accentuates noise of air movement

Nasal intubation is ideally performed with an endoscopic technique, as many indications for its use are better assessed by an endoscopic view of the airway. Do not blindly intubate if there is laryngotracheal pathology. In addition to standard endoscopes, there is now a single-use intubating endoscope, the Ambu® aScope™.

There are two general approaches: 1) Scope first—Tube is loaded at the base of the scope, which then navigates nares to trachea; 2) Tube first—Tube is placed blindly to a depth of 12–14cm in nares; the scope is then inserted through the tube to the larynx and into the trachea, then the tube is slid off. Tube first is faster, with less navigation.

Incrementalized
Blind Nasal Intubation

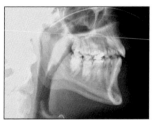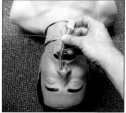

Left: *Insertion of the trumpet or tube into the naris initially straight back, perpendicular to the face, and medial toward the septum. Radiograph shows the tube in the nasopharynx.*

Right: *Advance the tracheal tube toward the larynx, while keeping the base of the tube directed at the contralateral nipple. This keeps the tube midline as it passes toward the larynx.*

Incrementalized Nasal Intubation Technique (S-T-S-T-S-T): Spray, Trumpet, Spray, Tube, Spray, Tube.

1. **S:** Spray anesthetic and vasoconstrictant into nares (combination of oxymetazoline and 4% topical lidocaine).

2. **T:** Insert 32 French soft nasal trumpet, lubricated with 2% lidocaine jelly, straight back (90° to face plane), directed midline.

3. **S:** Spray anesthetic through the trumpet twice. Patient will cough as anesthesia hits the larynx. Remove the trumpet.

4. **T:** Insert the tracheal tube to approximately 12–14cm, keeping the proximal end of the tube directed toward the patient's contralateral nipple (this directs the tip of the tube toward the midline, as shown above). Loud breath sounds should be audible through the tube.

5. **S:** Spray anesthetic once more through the tracheal tube.

6. **T:** Pass the tracheal tube through the cords on inspiration.

7. Confirm placement (loss of phonation, breath sounds, end-tidal CO_2) and secure the tube (26cm at naris for women, 28cm for men).

Nasal Intubation
with Endoscopic Guidance

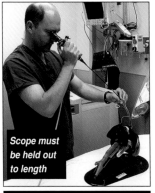

Scope must be held out to length

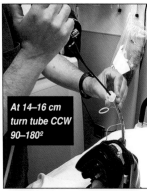

At 14–16 cm turn tube CCW 90–180º

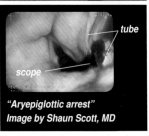

tube

scope

"Aryepiglottic arrest"
Image by Shaun Scott, MD

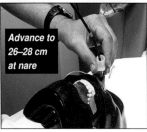

Advance to 26–28 cm at nare

Sequence of nasotracheal endoscopic intubation, using a "tube first" approach. Tube has been placed in nare to depth of 12–14 cm (top left), followed by endoscopic navigation into trachea—to level of carina—and then is slid off the scope using a CCW turn (top right) to depth of 26–28 cm (bottom right).

A tube-first approcah minimizes endoscopic navigation. Use topicalization and nasal trumpet, and ideally have the patient as upright as possible.

Oral Endoscopic Intubation

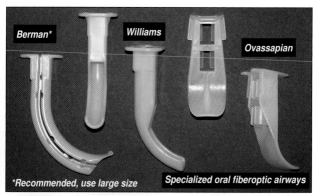

Berman*

Williams

Ovassapian

*Recommended, use large size

Specialized oral fiberoptic airways

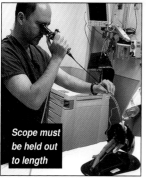

Scope must be held out to length

Oral endoscopic intubation has a shorter distance but a more acute angle than nasal.

The scope must navigate the curve of the tongue and through the gap between the tongue and posterior pharynx. The view on exiting the oral airway may be poor. Specialized airways help get around angle of the mouth.

Intubation via the oral route can be very challenging in supine patients with poor muscular tone. Lift the mandible (with jaw thrust or laryngoscope), and lift up on the oral airway to open the hypopharyngeal space. Once the larynx is seen, advance the scope to the carina, and then pass the tube off the scope with CCW rotation. LMA devices overcome many technical issues of oral endoscopy.

Save a Life—Cut the Neck!

The surgical airway has been wrongly termed "the failed airway." It should be "the surgically inevitable airway," to clearly label it as something that needed to happen and was going to happen at some point in the patient's care. When rescue oxygenation via passive oxygenation, face mask, and supraglottic airways will not work, and the patient cannot be intubated from above — we must cut the neck to save a life.

The first response to hypoxia (and inability to intubate) should not be to cut the neck — but rather to oxygenate — via the incrementalized approach and using SGAs as needed. If oxygenation will not work, however, providers must be pro-active and start the surgical airway early — as time to ventilation is approximately 100 seconds.

Major facial trauma, dynamic pathology about the base of tongue and mouth, and massive fluids (from below) commonly preclude oxygenation and require surgical airways.

An incrementalized approach to the surgical airway includes:
- Move to the side of the patient that matches your dominant hand.
- Position patient 45 degrees head up, with neck extension.
- Continue oxygenation/ventilation efforts during the procedure.
- Find landmarks via "laryngeal handshake."
- Stabilize the larynx with your non-dominant hand.
- Use sternal stabilization to make a vertical incision.
- Vertical incision should be 2.5–3 fingers length, from mid thyroid down.
- Verify the cricothyroid membrane with your non-dominant index finger.
- Cut horizontally through CTM, finger feels cartilaginous cage.
- Insert the tube, check depth/CO2, secure the tube, CXR.

Surgical Airway Anatomy

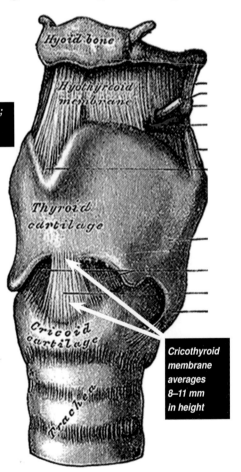

Hyoid bone

Hyothyroid membrane

Male larynx; prominent thyroid

Thyroid cartilage

Thyroid overlaps cricoid laterally

Cricoid cartilage

Cricothyroid membrane averages 8–11 mm in height

Trachea

Surgical Airway Anatomy

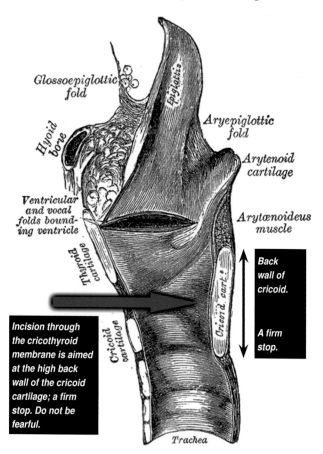

Glossoepiglottic fold

Epiglottis

Aryepiglottic fold

Hyoid bone

Arytenoid cartilage

Ventricular and vocal folds bounding ventricle

Arytænoideus muscle

Thyroid cartilage

Cricoid cartil.

Back wall of cricoid.

A firm stop.

Incision through the cricothyroid membrane is aimed at the high back wall of the cricoid cartilage; a firm stop. Do not be fearful.

Cricoid cartilage

Trachea

Surgical Airway Anatomy
The Cartilaginous Cage

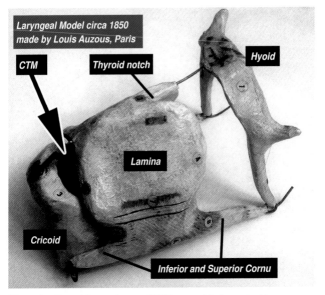

Laryngeal Model circa 1850 made by Louis Auzous, Paris

CTM

Thyroid notch

Hyoid

Lamina

Cricoid

Inferior and Superior Cornu

The cricothyroid membrane (CTM, arrow) is bounded by a "cartilaginous cage" that is made up of the thyroid cartilage (above the CTM), the anterior cricoid ring (below), the overlap of the thyroid on top of the cricoid (laterally) and the high back wall of the cricoid cartilage (not shown above; see page 106).

The inferior thyroid cornu overlaps the cricoid cartilage on either side. The superior cornu extend almost to hyoid bone. This is a male thyroid—prominent notch and acute angle of lamina.

Surgical Airway Anatomy
The Cartilaginous Cage

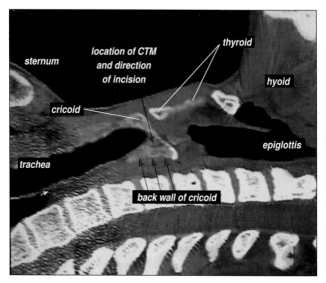

CT imaging of the neck in a sagittal orientation shows critical landmarks and demonstrates the cartilaginous cage.
Emergency providers who order and review lots of CT neck studies should use this modality to master laryngeal anatomy.

Notice the proximity of the back wall of the cricoid to the spine. A tracheal hook is necessary when performing a tracheostomy, but the larynx will not "drop" backward during a cricothyrotomy. A hook is not necessary to hold the larynx.

The author advocates scalpel-finger-tube technique for cricothyrotomy; as shown on p. 111–113.

Laryngeal Handshake
Rock the Rhomboid

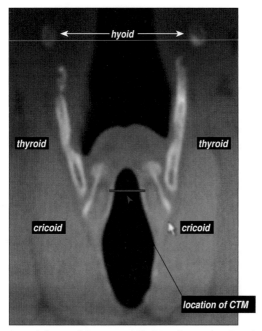

CT imaging of the neck in a coronal view shows the rhomboid arrangement of the laryngeal structures.

The superior cornu of the thyroid almost reaches the hyoid.

The inferior cornu of the thyroid overlaps the cricoid cartilage. This is important, because it limits the lateral movement of a scalpel as the CTM membrane is incised (ie, don't worry about going too lateral, since there is a firm lateral stop created by overlapping thyroid).

Laryngeal Handshake

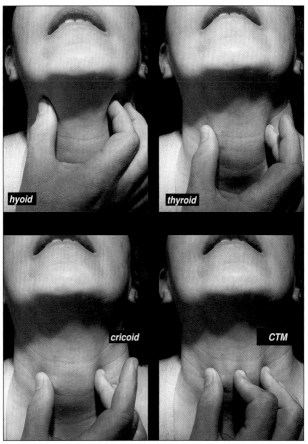

The "laryngeal handshake" uses 5 fingers to "rock the rhomboid" of the larynx and palpate from top to bottom: hyoid-thyroid-cricoid.

Incrementalized Approach to Cricothyrotomy

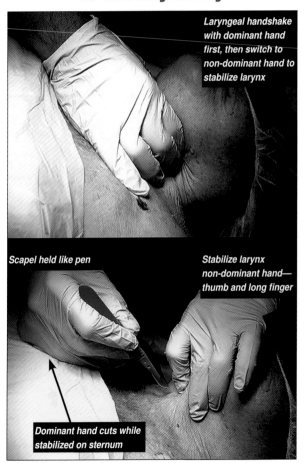

Laryngeal handshake with dominant hand first, then switch to non-dominant hand to stabilize larynx

Scapel held like pen

Stabilize larynx non-dominant hand— thumb and long finger

Dominant hand cuts while stabilized on sternum

Incrementalized Approach to Cricothyrotomy

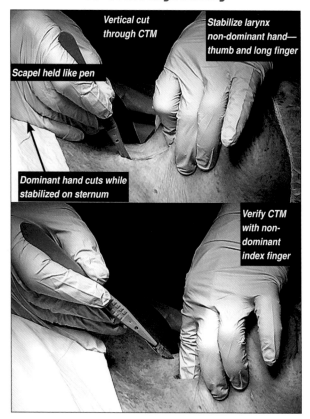

Vertical cut through CTM

Stabilize larynx non-dominant hand—thumb and long finger

Scapel held like pen

Dominant hand cuts while stabilized on sternum

Verify CTM with non-dominant index finger

Incrementalized Approach to Cricothyrotomy

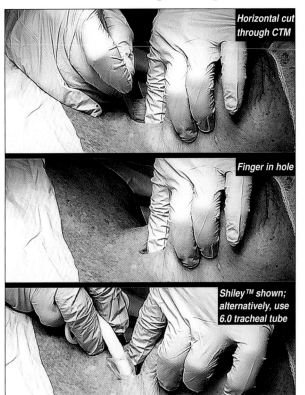

Horizontal cut through CTM

Finger in hole

Shiley™ shown; alternatively, use 6.0 tracheal tube

Cricothyrotomy
Tube Considerations

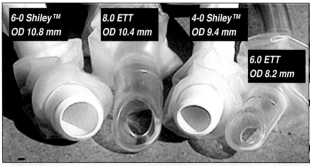

6-0 Shiley™
OD 10.8 mm

8.0 ETT
OD 10.4 mm

4-0 Shiley™
OD 9.4 mm

6.0 ETT
OD 8.2 mm

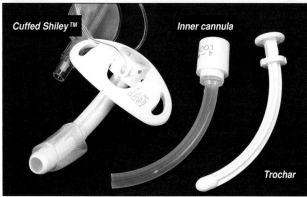

Cuffed Shiley™

Inner cannula

Trochar

Many different tubes and tracheostomy devices can be placed through the cricothyroid membrane, but operators should know their outer diameters, given the relatively small size of the cricothyroid membrane (8–11 mm; smaller in females, larger in males). Shiley™ tracheostomy tubes (bottom photo) have an inner cannula (needed for ventilation) and a trochar (for insertion).

Surgical Airways
Post Procedure Concerns and Tracheostomy Tube Management

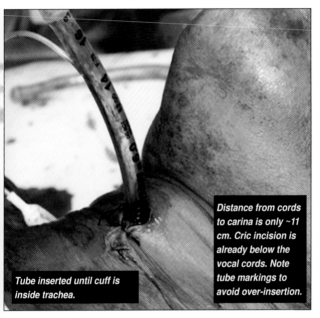

Distance from cords to carina is only ~11 cm. Cric incision is already below the vocal cords. Note tube markings to avoid over-insertion.

Tube inserted until cuff is inside trachea.

Air movement through the tube will be evident in a spontaneously breathing patient. Verify end-tidal CO_2 if you have any concern, and listen for symmetric breath sounds. It is common to over-insert a tracheal tube, which can cause hyperinflation of a lung and tracheal shift (mistakenly suggesting pneumothorax).

Pneumothorax is not uncommon after an emergent surgical airway because air can dissect down from the surgical incision.

References

Weingart SD, Levitan RM. Preoxygenation and Prevention of Desaturation During Emergency Airway Management. *Ann Emerg Med.* 2012;59(3):165–75.

Levitan RM, Kovacs G. "Direct Laryngoscopy" in Hung & Murphy's Management of the Difficult and Failed Airway, 2e, McGraw Hill, New York, 2012.

Levitan RM, Heitz JW, Sweeney M, Cooper RM. The Complexities of Tracheal Intubation With Direct Laryngoscopy and Alternative Intubation Devices. *Ann Emerg Med.* 2011;57:240–7.

Levitan RM, Everett WW, Kinkle WC, Levin WJ. Laryngeal View During Laryngoscopy: A Randomized Trial Comparing Cricoid Pressure, BURP, and Bimanual Laryngoscopy. *Ann Emerg Med.* 2006;47:548–55.

Collins JS, Lemmens HJ, Brodsky JB, Brock-Utne JG, Levitan RM. Laryngoscopy and morbid obesity: a comparison of the "sniff" and "ramped" positions. **Obes Surg.** 2004;14:1171–5.

Levitan RM. Patient safety in emergency airway management and rapid sequence intubation: metaphorical lessons from skydiving. *Ann Emerg Med.* 2003;42:81–7.

Levitan RM, Mechem CC, Ochroch EA, Shofer FS, Hollander JE. Head Elevated Laryngoscopy Positioning (HELP): Improving laryngeal exposure during laryngoscopy by increasing head elevation. *Ann Emerg Med.* 2003;41:322–30.

Online Resources

Airway Cam videos — **airwaycam.com/videos**

Academic Life in Emergency Medicine, Michele Lin — **aliem.com**

Jim Ducanto & Yen Chow — **vimeo.com/airwaynautics**

Airway Interventions and Management in Emergencies.
George Kovacs, Adam Law — **aimeairway.ca**

Bronchoscopy Atlas — **bronchoscopy.org**

Difficult Airway Society, UK — **das.uk.com**

Emergency Medicine Cases. Anton Helman —
emergencymedicinecases.com/category/podcast/best-case-ever

Emergency Medicine & Critcal Care. Scott Weingart — **emcrit.org**

Reuben Strayer — **emupdates.com**

Oli Flower & Roger Harris, et al. — **intensivecarenetwork.com**

Mike Cadogan & Chris Nickson — **lifeinthefastlane.com**

Pediatric Emergency Medicine an Educational and Directional Podcast.
Andy Sloas — **pemed.org**

Pre-Hospital & Retrieval Medicine, Minh Le Cong —
prehospitalmed.com

Resuscitationist's Awesome Guide to Everything. Chris Nickson,
Cliff Reid, Haney Mallemat, Michaela Cartner, Karel Habig —
ragepodcast.com

Rezaie's Evidence Based Evaluation of Literature. Salim Rezale,
Matt Austin, Anand Swaminathan — **rebelem.com**

Resuscitation Medicine Education, Cliff Reid — **resus.me**

Social Media & Critical Care Conference —
smacc.net.au/about-us/welcome

Society Airway Management, US — **samhq.com**

Notes

Notes

Pre-Oxygenation, Positioning, Preparation

1. Cardiac arrest or near arrest?	
SGA	**2. Obvious oral pathology** Mask and SGA impossible? →Nose or Neck
Oral Intubation	**3. Intrinsic** **Laryngo-tracheal pathology?** → Endoscopy-trach

4. Anatomic concerns?
Distortion
Dysproportion
Dentition
Dysmobility

5. Physiologic concerns?
Hemodynamics
Oxygenation
Ventilation

— — — — — — — RSI Line — — — — — — — —

Oral intubation (Direct, Video, or DL/VL)
with no DESAT (nasal cannula—apneic oxygenation)
Rescue Oxygenation (apneic oxygenation, SGA, BVM-PEEP)
Rescue Intubation (via SGA, surgical airway)

The decision to use muscle relaxants (crossing the RSI line – represented by dashes) is based on a redundancy of safety. If intubation fails after RSI, the patient will need to be oxygenated and ventilated.

In cardiac arrest the priority is oxygenation, speed, and not interrupting resuscitation.

With obvious anatomic pathology about the mouth, or laryngo-tracheal pathology, there is no redundancy of safety. Mask ventilation and supraglottic airways may not work. Rescue intubation in these situations involves a surgical airway (i.e., a cric or trach, depending on level of pathology). Muscle relaxants are generally avoided.

If intubation fails after crossing the RSI line, the priority is rescue oxygenation before rescue intubation.